THE REAL
SEXY
SMART
AND STRONG

30 tips to boost confidence, get fit and feel great, inside and out

DAVID PATCHELL-EVANS

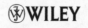

WILEY
John Wiley & Sons Canada, Ltd.

Library and Archives Canada Cataloguing in Publication

Patchell-Evans, David
 The real sexy, smart, and strong : living with confidence / David Patchell-Evans.
Includes index.
ISBN 978-0-470-16124-1
 1. Exercise. 2. Physical fitness. I. Title.
RA776.P375 2009   613.7   C2009-902274-5

Production Credits
Cover Design: Ian Koo
Interior Design: Michael Chan
Printer: Tri-graphic

Editorial Credits
Editor: Leah Fairbank
Project Coordinator: Pauline Ricablanca

John Wiley & Sons Canada, Ltd.
6045 Freemont Blvd.
Mississauga, Ontario
L5R 4J3

Printed in Canada

1 2 3 4 5 TRI 13 12 11 10 09

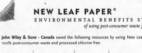

NEW LEAF PAPER®
ENVIRONMENTAL BENEFITS STATEMENT
of using post-consumer waste fiber vs. virgin fiber

John Wiley & Sons - Canada saved the following resources by using New Leaf Pioneer, made with 100% post-consumer waste and processed chlorine free:

trees	water	energy	solid waste	greenhouse gases
218 fully grown	93,836 gallons	158 million Btu	10,467 pounds	20,622 pounds

Calculations based on research by Environmental Defense Fund and other members of the Paper Task Force.

www.newleafpaper.com

ANCIENT FOREST FRIENDLY™

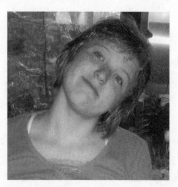

This book is dedicated to every autistic child; to every autistic adult and to all the families that love and support them.

A special dedication to my equally special daughter Tygre, who does not have autism. Who does have concern, caring and love for her sister and dad in her heart and soul. Tygre who lives every day with a smile, friendliness and compassion for others. Tygre, your dancing feet and dancing heart are a wonderful example for me.

I love you both.

Daddy

All proceeds from this book will support important research by the Kilee Patchell-Evans Autism Research Group, based in Canada, into the cause and cure for autism.

CONTENTS

by Peggy McColl, *New York Times* bestselling author of
Your Destiny Switch

When it comes to health and happiness, David Patchell-Evans ("Patch") and I speak the same language. As a worldwide teacher of empowerment, positive attitude, and emotional mastery, my life's work involves helping people discover their best self—their *real* self. Feeling more vital, more comfortable in your own skin, smarter, more productive, and stronger are *huge* factors in achieving success in life. Patch and I share this mission of inspiring people to rev up their lives, to live with passion, energy, health and joy—and showing them how to do it.

When I first met Patch a few years ago, I was deeply impressed by his unwavering commitment to empowering people through regular physical activity and positive attitude. He is not afraid to share the hopes, dreams, achievements, setbacks, challenges and victories in his own life to show you that you don't have to be perfect. Patch gets you to focus on what you *can* do, not on what you *can't* do. He guides you every step of the way. Everything Patch suggests in this book, he himself has done, over and over again. When it comes to fitness, he is the "real deal."

The guiding force of Patch's life is the leadership he shows in motivating hundreds of thousands of people all over the world to create high levels of health and well-being in their day-to-day lives. He very aptly calls this book "The Real Sexy Smart and Strong" with emphasis on the *real*. Rather than approach fitness as a discipline in which we have to push our body to unrealistic lengths, instead Patch gives us the powerful and comforting insight that fitness is really very easy and that you, and I, and virtually everyone we know—all of us—are capable of living our lives feeling sexy, smart, and strong. It doesn't take hours and hours every week. All it takes is twenty to thirty minutes three times a week.

In the pages of this book, Patch's encouraging words will convince you that you *can* make regular exercise part of your life and that the dividends you gain will be absolutely priceless.

Exercise has an impact on every part of our life. It improves our moods. It makes us more productive at work and at home. It gives us the stamina to withstand any stress, and indeed exercise is the number one stress-buster. It boosts our positive attitude and increases our self-esteem. It makes our body strong and resilient. It gives us the twinkle in our eye, the bounce in our step, and the energy that carries us into every day with a sense of joy and anticipation.

Let Patch coach you, convince you, and move you into bringing physical activity into your life. Try just a few of the ideas in the book, or better yet, try them all! You'll experience so many positive changes in your life. Keep it up! You are the real sexy, smart, and strong!

IT BEGINS WITH YOUR BODY

I wrote this book to inspire you to reap the joyful benefits of physical movement. I want to share my passion for exercise, to tell you how in more than thirty years in the fitness industry I have seen thousands of people's lives transformed by regular physical activity.

I titled this book *The Real Sexy, Smart, and Strong* with emphasis on the *real*. So often we are seduced by media images of what "sexy" means and we are convinced that there is no way we could match them. In today's society, "smart" often means being clever rather than having the deep intelligence that resides in the harmony of mind and body. "Strong" has come to mean powerful—as in getting your own way—or it evokes images of bodybuilders. All these are just illusions. They distort what sexy, smart, and strong *really* are.

So in this book I want us to get real—to realize that sexy is about feeling at home in your body and being comfortable with who you are. Regular physical exercise plays a big role in giving you a comfortable body confidence. Smart is about having a high level of energy and awareness of how you live your life. Strong is about being the best you can be and having the strength to live each day without getting overtired and stressed. Exercise helps you do the things you want to do in your life without being held back.

If I could get only one message across to you, it would be this: there are no rights and wrongs about looking or feeling good. Media images should never be the barometer of what is possible for you. There is only what works for *you*. However, there is one requirement: you must participate. You must move. Use it or lose it still applies to your body!

There is something magical about exercise. As you give yourself the gift of physical activity and your body gets fit, you'll become more accepting of your body. You'll start to look good because you'll be projecting energy and confidence from within. You'll have the glow of well-being. People are going to find that very attractive. Physical activity is crucial to your overall health.

In contrast, think about how "off" you feel when you have a cold. Your energy is low. You become cranky and lethargic. You don't feel like socializing. Your productivity lessens.

Now think about how you feel as your cold starts to dwindle. Your mood improves. Your energy, drive, and ambition resurface. You sleep better. You connect with people more easily. You get more done. You're happier.

The same is true of becoming fit. When you don't exercise, your body is acting like it has a cold. The only difference is that you're *accustomed* to it. You have all the symptoms of sickness—aches, pains, and low energy—but think it's normal. You think that's the way it is. Well, it doesn't have to be that way at all; you can change right now!

I see exercise as a form of self-respect. If you look after yourself, it means you're capable—physically as well as emotionally. Your body is absolutely great. It can do wonders. Most of you can achieve a fitness and health level that can really surprise you. Not to mention the fact that your body wants physical activity so badly that it rewards you when you do it by making you look good and feel good. There isn't anything else you can spend your money on that does as much for you as regular physical activity.

There isn't a medication you can take, a jazzy car you can buy, makeup, clothes, jewelry, or shoes that will make you feel the way you do when your body is fit and healthy. Plus, exercise is easy. I'm going to show you just *how* easy.

INVEST IN THIRTY MINUTES, THREE TIMES A WEEK

Half an hour, three times a week—that's all it takes to become fit and healthy and to stay that way. Sounds too good to believe, doesn't it? I'll bet you've been told that if you're going to get into exercising, you really have to "apply yourself" before you see any results. Most people think that means spending hours every week on some exercise machine or lifting weights.

The truth is that if you spend only thirty minutes, three times a week, doing some kind of fitness activity—particularly a combination of stretching, strength training, and cardiovascular exercise that you enjoy—within six months you will be in better physical shape than 90 percent of the population. Fitness isn't hard. *It's easy.* What's *hard* is being *unfit*.

Here's some more news: fit is not about being athletic, it's about being healthy. It's not about perfection, it's about knowing that you have reached the level where, as I love to say, "good enough is good enough." Good enough is reached when you have found exercise that works for *you* and that makes you functionally strong. You'll start to notice that your physical strength helps you lift those bags of groceries, throw out the trash, or give your child a piggy back ride. It makes you want to go dancing late into the night and helps you wake up in the morning feeling ready to take on the day.

Getting fit will allow you, over time, to set a special goal for yourself. One goal for me was rafting down the Colorado River in the Grand Canyon and doing some climbing there. Running the river's rapids was a huge challenge. Rapids are what I would call "controlled danger." There's a sense of exhilaration and excitement. Because I have rheumatoid arthritis, I'm less flexible than I was years ago, but, man, it was a wonderful feeling to be carried on the "roller coaster" of those rapids!

I also went out for a climb on the rocks—twenty-five minutes to climb and twenty-five minutes to get back. I jumped from rock to rock. In climbing slang, they call this "scrambling." When you're climbing, you can't think about what's below; you keep looking up and visualizing what it would be like to reach the top. This actually became a teaching for me for my life—no matter how precarious things look, don't look back, just keep going. Balance yourself forward. Tilt those loose rocks of life in the direction you want to go.

The really neat thing about this kind of experience is that it's immediate. You have to constantly make a choice about what your body is capable of. It is very much in the *now*. I have learned a lot from being in natural areas where my survival depends on keeping my wits about me and relying upon the strength reserves of my body and mind. When you do the climb and return again, it's an amazing feeling. For you, when you do something physical you have always wanted to do, I think you'll feel this same amazement. For many people, that satisfaction comes from doing any exercise at all: you will say to yourself, "*Wow, that was me! I did that.*"

Regular physical activity allows you to inhabit your body completely—to feel your muscles and organs, the air on your skin, the beating of your heart, your lungs full of oxygen. Many of us only pay attention to our bodies when something goes wrong—when we're sick or injured. Physical activity makes you *live in* and enjoy your body.

One of the key things that having arthritis has taught me is to focus on what *does* work. The GoodLife company I founded embraces the slogan "Don't let the things you can't do stop you from doing the things you can." A good friend of mine, Augie Nieto, has amyotrophic lateral sclerosis (ALS, or Lou Gehrig's disease). He says, "I wake up every morning and redefine normal. I don't mourn what

I can't do, I celebrate what I can do! I have a gift. I get to see the kindness of others every day."

Cherish each day how wonderful your body is and learn to care for it. Your body is made for activity. It craves movement. In fact, it needs exercise every forty-eight hours just to recover from the stresses of everyday life. It needs exercise to maintain strong bones and good skin, to lower your heart rate and unclog your arteries. It needs movement so that your life feels more zestful. A person who lives with zest, with oomph, is sexy, smart, and strong!

EMBRACE CHALLENGES AND DON'T HOLD BACK

In this book, I point out all the ways that exercise can improve your life. Every one of us has different challenges, situations that stress us, change us, and put us up against a wall. I know beyond any doubt that when your body is given all the opportunities to enjoy its natural capacity for movement, the energy reserves you build up help you cope with what life throws your way. In fact, it helps you do *more* than cope—it helps you *thrive*.

I call my own personal challenges the three A's—the three things that shaped my life.

The first A is an accident I had at age nineteen. I broke and tore apart my right arm, shoulder, and chest while riding a motorcycle. I was temporarily paralyzed and spent six months in rehabilitation. Exercise played a huge role in my recovery. At the Fowler Kennedy Sport Medicine Clinic in London, Ontario, I worked alongside both elite athletes who were training and regular folks who had been injured. This is when I first discovered my passion for making people feel better through physical activity because I experienced firsthand how it made *me* and all the other participants in the clinic feel better too. If I hadn't had that accident, I might not have become a fitness professional and club owner. I might not have grown my company to more than 170 clubs with more than 500,000 members. I might not have gone all over the world speaking about fitness.

The second A is arthritis. At age thirty-two, I woke up one morning, instantly crippled. My whole body was swollen, inflamed and in total pain. I was diagnosed with rheumatoid arthritis. I had been an elite athlete, a five-time rowing champion, and overnight I couldn't even turn a doorknob. When I first tried to go back to exercising, I actually had to have someone spin the wheels of the stationary exercise bike for me. That was quite a blow to the guy who people thought of as Mr. GoodLife Fitness. I used exercise to help me mentally cope with the symptoms and to regain physical strength and mobility. To this day, exercise helps me control the arthritis. I get into more detail about my arthritis in Chapter 28: Exercising with Chronic Pain.

The third A is autism. At the age of two and a half, my eldest daughter, Kilee, started showing marked changes in behavior. Her kisses turned into biting, her laughter into constant screams. She started pushing me away when I tried to hug her. She wouldn't make eye contact. She seemed lost in her own world. I went through a bewildering journey of trying to figure out what was going on. I still remember the initial devastation I felt upon hearing a doctor say, "Your daughter is autistic."

I became determined to help Kilee become the best she could be. I chose not to focus on her condition but on her potential. I chose to love her unconditionally. All my energy went into a very intensive home learning program for her, aimed at drawing the best out of her. It's been hard, as her form of autism is fairly severe. Yet she has made enormous strides—in using basic words, socializing, and playing sports. I also made the decision to commit myself to finding the cure for autism. I've provided the initial funding for an innovative research program under the direction of neuroscientist Dr. Derrick MacFabe at the University of Western Ontario in London, Ontario. I con-

tinue to support that program, closing in on $3 million
I've donated to the research team. The researchers have
made some intriguing discoveries, giving them important
clues about the possible cause of autism. They've published several papers that have drawn international attention and Dr. MacFabe is speaking all over the world about
his findings. In fact, I was awarded the Medal of Honour
by the Canadian Medical Association for my role. All the
proceeds of this book are going to autism research to help
find a cure for this condition that affects one in every 150
children worldwide.

You might ask what physical activity has to do with my
journey as a parent of an autistic child. The answer is
twofold. By keeping up my own regular physical activity,
my energy levels stay high, my mind stays sharp, and I
cope better with stress—and raising an autistic child can
be very stressful. Secondly, I have involved regular physical activity in Kilee's treatment program, with the result
that today she has a high level of physical skill. She swims,
skis, bikes, runs, and rides horseback. She's thirteen now,
and I am starting her at one of my fitness clubs. Being
physically active has helped her to improve both her
cognitive and emotional strength. It allows her to interact
socially even though she uses few words: in movement
she is an equal.

My three A's have given me a sensitivity toward people whose bodies are not perfect, people who have had injuries and accidents, people who are coping with chronic conditions such as arthritis or diabetes or who are recovering from a heart attack or stroke, and also people who are overwhelmed or scared to exercise because of inexperience. I know what someone means when he or she says, "I had this horrible injury and I feel like I can't do things." I can give people the reassurance that there *are* things they can do and that their body can indeed find a movement level that will help them.

What are your own personal challenges, and how might physical activity help you? Exercise influences the biggest A of all—your attitude. When life hits you broadside, respond with your big A, your attitude. And follow your big A with the three E's: energy, excitement, and enthusiasm. Exercise helps you feel the three E's in the body. When you feel it in the body, you feel it in the mind, heart, and spirit. There is no split between mind and body—you are one whole human being.

STAYING MOTIVATED

I know there are going to be times when you will feel discouraged with exercising. Particularly if you've been sedentary for a long time and are just getting started with exercise, your subconscious mind (a creature of habit) is going to give you some mental push-back in the form of resistance. One of the major forms of resistance is discouragement. How can you regenerate your motivation?

This is how to get motivated. First, reflect on why you are exercising. What did you want for yourself when you first started? Did you want to lose weight? Did you want to make your muscles stronger? Did you want a better sex life? Did you want to walk around the block with your kids and not feel winded? Did you want to play with your grandkids? Did you want to go on a really active vacation with friends?

Sometimes discouragement morphs into a feeling of boredom. "This is too routine," you might complain. I often like to compare exercising to showering. Why do you shower regularly? So that your skin stays clean and you won't have BO! Is showering routine? Absolutely. You do it because you want to have healthy, clean skin and hair.

It's the same with exercise. You exercise because you want your body to be in good shape. You want good health, good strength. Yes, this will require a "routine" of physical activity. However, the great thing about exercise, unlike showering or brushing your teeth, is that there are so many variations of it. You can jog one day, go to the fitness club the next, work on the bicycle the next time, switch to the stair machine, choose a group fitness class, or go for a long walk. There are hundreds of choices!

Don't allow yourself to fall into the mindset of feeling discouraged. Find joy in the fact that by doing regular physical activity you will be healthier and happier. Regular doesn't have to mean boring. Regular just means that you're consistently investing your time and energy into being healthy—and that's nothing to be discouraged about!

UN-LIMIT YOURSELF

Most of the limitations you think you have are the ones *you* have decided on. They are often entirely self-imposed. You might think, "I can't do this, I can't do that, I would never do that, my parents could never do that, I never played baseball, I've never climbed a mountain, I never, never, never … "—it's the old broken record in your head. Throw out that negative thinking right now! Learn to play a positive message in your head because it's all about attitude. After all, you are becoming the *real* sexy, smart, and strong!

Most of us sell ourselves short. We think that because we're aging, or we were no good in physical education class at school, or we're too short, too tall, too skinny, too fat, etc., that we are limited. When we let these limitations dictate our reality, we compromise our quality of life.

Sure, in one sense we all have some limitations. Everyone's body is different. People have differing abilities. However, we give ourselves far too little credit for the fact that very often we *can* go beyond our perceived limitations. We've set the bar too low in our lives.

Stories abound about everyday people accomplishing amazing feats. A visually impaired person has climbed Mount Everest! Special needs individuals excel in the Special Olympics. I have had the good fortune to meet Silken Laumann and Rick Hansen. Silken, a four-time Olympian rower, was favored to win a gold medal at the 1992 Olympics. In rowing practice, her shell was accidentally rammed hard by another boat, ripping apart the muscles of one leg. After five surgeries, skin grafts, and the removal of hundreds of wood splinters, she went on to compete again, capturing an Olympic bronze medal just ten weeks later.

Rick Hansen lost the use of his legs after a car crash paralyzed him at age fifteen. He graduated with a physical education degree—the first student with a disability to do so. In 1985 he began his "Man In Motion" journey in a wheelchair around the whole world to raise money for spinal cord injuries, covering almost 25,000 miles (40,000 kilometers) across thirty-four countries. When you meet Silken and Rick, you come to understand that you have no limits.

One of my absolute favorite stories is about Roger Bannister, the first man to run the four-minute mile. Prior to Bannister running the four-minute mile, everyone, including the medical professionals, said it couldn't be done. Bannister was told that if he ran a four-minute mile, his head would explode. So when he finished the race on May 6, 1954, in Oxford, England, he fell to the ground, holding his head between his hands. When asked why, the story goes that he said, "I thought my head might blow up." The point is, he did it anyway. He believed in himself and in possibilities. And since he did it, numerous other runners have done it as well.

Many of us spend our adult years shrinking into our limitations rather than expanding into our potential. Fitness is one way to reverse that kind of thinking. When you begin to empower your body to feel stronger and healthier, you will begin to feel more empowered in *all* areas of your life. That's why there's a link between fitness and mood, and between fitness and productivity, which I'll discuss in detail in Chapter 8: A Natural Treatment for Depression and Chapter 9: Keep Your Brain on Exercise.

It's all up to you. Anyone can achieve a higher quality of life if he or she wants it. Exercise will help you live longer, feel better, and accomplish more. Choose to become one of the un-limited. Choose to be the real sexy, smart, and strong!

YOU REALLY CAN BE SEXY, SMART, AND STRONG

Every time you go for a walk or a run, go out dancing with friends, swim, cross-country ski, in fact do anything physical at all, you are positively influencing your ability to feel good.

Many people begin exercising because they are unhappy with their weight—they don't like their legs, belly, arms, or think they should be more muscular. Others want to improve their sex lives or skin, or they want to have more energy—there are a million reasons to start exercising, and we will explore many of them in Part I.

Let's clear one thing up from the get-go: I have never met a person who thinks he or she has a perfect body—and that's actually a good thing, because getting into shape is not about attaining perfection. Perfection is an illusion!

This book is about being *real* and becoming the very best you can be. *Best never means perfect.*

When you exercise, you will feel the vitality and energy in *your own body.* Exercise can give you an inner and outer radiance that makes people notice you. You'll look good by looking like *you* at your very best, by feeling right inside your skin and heightening your aliveness as a human being!

In Part I, we'll explore all the reasons for beginning an exercise program. We'll learn about endorphins, those wonderful brain chemicals released during exercise that make you feel so good. We'll talk about the effect of exercise on longevity and on the health of your heart and lungs. You'll find out how exercise improves your sex life, protects you from burnout, and elevates your mood.

When you get fit, you gradually transform yourself into more of who you want to be. Your muscles feel firmer. You hold your head a little higher. Your joints are aligned. Your skin starts to look better. Your breathing improves. You eliminate toxins or bad chemicals from your body. You sleep better. You think more clearly. You have more fun! If you activate your endorphins every day, you're going to start feeling and thinking, "Wow, life is great!" To most people, radiating that kind of attitude is sexy!

CHAPTER 1

LIVE LONGER

In 2009 scientists all over the world celebrated the two hundredth anniversary of Charles Darwin's birth. When we think of Darwin, the famous phrase *survival of the fittest* comes to mind. We know he was referring to evolution; however, I can't help but interpret *survival of the fittest* in the context of physical fitness: *We are more likely to survive longer if we are fit.*

Major proof of this is found in the well-known Framingham Heart Study, considered one of the most definitive studies of heart health. Starting in 1948, researchers followed more than five thousand men and women in Framingham, Massachusetts, for a forty-year period. The study proved that those who exercised regularly, ranging from a moderate to more intense level, lived from 1.5 to 3.7 years longer than those who didn't exercise.

Did you know?

One of the ways physicians predict your physiological "age" is by conducting stress tests on a treadmill. You begin by walking at an easy pace. After a few minutes, the incline and speed are increased to intensify the workload on your heart and lungs in order to measure your physical working capacity. Performing well on the stress test indicates that your heart and lungs are in good shape and working well, which is a major factor in increasing your life expectancy!

I am the chairperson of the board of directors for the International Health, Racquet & Sportsclub Association (IHRSA), the largest fitness association in the world. IHRSA represents 9,100 fitness and health facilities in more than 78 countries, a staggering total of more than 100 million club members. This gives me a global perspective about fitness. It is our conviction that *working out a few times a week can add as many as* nine years *to your life*, far more than the one to three years reported by the Framingham study.

Take, for example, a report published in 2008 in the *Archives of Internal Medicine* that looked at parts of DNA known as telomeres. Telomeres are the protective ends of your chromosomes and are believed to help prevent cell damage. They grow shorter as you age, and so the longer the time during your lifespan that telomeres can keep their length, the better. Researchers studied the effect of exercise on the length of telomeres by comparing more than twelve hundred sets of identical twins and their exercise habits. In each set, the twin who exercised regularly maintained significantly longer telomeres, making him or her physiologically nine years younger than the more sedentary identical sibling, whose telomeres had shortened (in other words, the sedentary twin was not maintaining enough telomere protection).

Being physically active has also been proven to reduce the risk of heart disease, stroke, and many types of cancer; lower blood pressure; make weight control easier; and improve your overall quality of life. By preventing these lifestyle diseases, or delaying their onset, you'll have a longer, better life.

DO THIS

List five benefits of exercise I mentioned in this chapter. Think of some specific physical activities that could help you get these results. Choose the activity you like best from your list. And then this week, do it!

CHAPTER 2

TURN ON THOSE ENDORPHINS

Have you ever noticed how exuberant you feel after chasing your kids around the yard or a night of dancing? That's because you body's endorphins are working!

Endorphins are the brain chemicals that make you feel good—and they are turned on by physical activity. They are produced in every cell of your body. They belong to a family of chemicals (called neuropeptides) and hormones that help relax body tissue and ease pain (they are often called nature's morphine). These wonderful pleasure boosters respond to physical movement and don't cost you a dime!

Did you know?

Even ten minutes of moderately vigorous exercise (producing a pulse rate of 80 to 120 beats per minute, depending on your age and fitness level) can raise your endorphin levels for one hour.

The good thing is that they're a positive and healthy "addiction." Once your body gets used to feeling the natural pleasure of exercise, your brain chemicals urge you to want more! And what's the effect of that? You begin to crave exercise! You know how delicious a piece of chocolate tastes? Well, when your body really starts feeling the benefits of exercise, you'll be looking forward to your regular exercise times to give you those "delicious" endorphins—something to savor indeed.

DO THIS

Every time you finish a physical activity, take a moment to notice how good you feel. At least once or twice a week, do something to deliberately wake up your endorphins. Go for a brisk walk somewhere beautiful. Play outside with your kids or your pet. When no one is home, put on your favorite music and dance around.

CHAPTER 3

COME ON, BABY, LIGHT MY FIRE

What's a secret reason a lot of people work out? You guessed it. It's the mating game.

Simply put, if you work out on a regular basis, you'll find that a very positive spin-off may well be that your sex life improves. Like that's a big surprise! A recent study of middle-aged males found that those who worked out regularly were far less likely to experience erectile dysfunction or to require the help of a drug such as Viagra. Why? Because exercise improves circulation of blood to all body parts. Everything works better, and the same thing happens for women.

Did you know?

The Harvard School of Public Health reports that a study involving more than thirty-one thousand men revealed that men who are physically active are 30 percent less likely to experience erectile dysfunction than men with little or no physical activity.

Another study at the University of British Columbia found that twenty minutes of exercise spurred greater sexual response in the women participants compared to those who hadn't exercised.

Why does exercise seem to have such a beneficial effect on our libidos? From a psychological standpoint, our self-esteem increases as we become more fit and comfortable in our bodies, which means we are more open to giving and receiving pleasure. From a physiological standpoint, if you have better blood flow, your whole body will be more sensitive and responsive. Just as your heart works better if it has a good blood flow, so does the rest of you! You get the point ...

Remember those endorphins I told you about? Well, good sex releases endorphins too! The endorphins that make you feel good during exercise also encourage you to want to feel good in other ways.

Not to mention the fact that *being in good shape means you can sustain your sexual activity for a much longer period of time and with greater frequency over your entire life.* Desire is heightened too, and physical recovery (such as returning your heart rate to normal) is quicker. Twenty- to thirty-minute strength training workouts a couple times a week help men and women maintain good levels of testosterone, which is key to your sex drive. To top it all off, by staying in shape you will extend your active sex life into your seventies, eighties, or even nineties. Here's a bonus—your sexual activities can become exercise, too (just use your imagination!). Sex reduces stress. Sex can even help you burn calories. Sound good?

DO THIS

Make a list of four people you know whom you consider sexy. Now add number five to the list: you. You're in great company! Make a coffee date with each of the four, and ask them what they do to stay in shape and what the source of their boundless energy is. Be prepared to get inspired. Can you do those things too? I bet you can!

CHAPTER 4
YOUR BODY'S BIGGEST ORGAN

Many people don't realize that exercise is not just about getting great muscles, more strength, and a healthy heart and lungs. It's also about making your body's biggest organ—your skin—look fantastic. Yes, your skin really is the largest organ of your body, although we don't often think of it that way.

Exercise increases circulation and delivers important nutrients to your skin, helping you get rid of toxins. It also helps your body produce natural collagen, the fibers in your skin that slow down aging and prevent wrinkles. As a result, people who exercise have better complexions. Beauty products, lotions, and cleansers might help, but they won't bring about the inside-out change you need for truly healthy skin. By giving your skin what it needs through regular physical activity, you're going to look younger and more vibrant.

Another benefit of exercise is that it helps you relax by combating the effects of stress—which in turn relaxes your face muscles! This means that your wrinkles will begin to soften. You may not be able to prevent every crow's foot from forming as you age (and why would you want to?), but you'll certainly be able to slow them down.

The process that makes your skin healthy also makes your hair healthier, shinier, and more durable because a vigorous body with a healthy blood flow will encourage the growth of your hair. (And if you're genetically susceptible to male pattern baldness, you can take comfort in the fact that the top of your head will have the same healthy complexion as the rest of you!)

A great complexion and shiny hair—I don't know about you, but to me these are sexy!

KEEP YOUR SKIN HYDRATED
Don't forget the role that water plays in keeping your skin looking young and fresh and in maintaining your overall health. Statistics show that 75 percent of North Americans are borderline dehydrated and more than one-third of North Americans have a weak thirst instinct, which means that we often eat when we should be drinking water. This could explain why so many of us have an impulse to snack and take in unnecessary calories.

Did you know?

Some medical professionals say that adequate water intake can have an effect on easing back and joint pain.

Even very mild dehydration will make your skin dryer, which makes your face look taut and older. It can also slow down your metabolism by as much as 3 percent. Lack of water is the number-one cause of daytime fatigue, so if you're feeling tired at midday, don't reach for a sugary soft drink—empty calories and the carbonation process actually contribute to increasing thirst and dryness in your skin. Forget caffeine too! Caffeine gives you an energy buzz but is also dehydrating. (And the energy high you get is rapidly followed by an energy low.)

I'm not suggesting you should never drink a soda. Nor do I mean that you have to forgo your favorite latte. I'm just cautioning that if sodas and coffee are currently your beverages of choice, you will look and feel much better if you add more fresh water into your diet.

DO THIS

Divert some of this month's "beauty budget" into an exercise budget. Your body's biggest organ will thank you.

CHAPTER 5

STAND TALL

Have you ever noticed how tall a dancer looks, even if she's only five-foot-three (160 centimeters)? It's because of the way she holds her body—her spine is long, her shoulders open, her head held high. All kinds of self-help books teach you that confidence is an attitude—and it is. But it's not just about your state of mind; it's also about your body. Did you know that *you can alter your level of self-assurance simply by standing taller?*

Unfortunately, because we spend too much time hunched over desks at computers, slouching in chairs, and lounging on the couch, most people have bad posture. Many adolescents forgo exercise in favor of video games. If you want great posture, you have to exercise! Your body needs muscular strength to hold you upright. This is especially true as you age. You don't have to succumb to stooping as you grow older. If you do regular physical activity, you can walk as tall at eighty as you did at eighteen. Exercise will give you muscle definition, and firm muscles help you look good at any age!

Did you know?

Regular weight-bearing exercise not only strengthens the muscles of your back, but it strengthens your bones as well. Physical activity helps maintain bone density, which is important in preventing osteoporosis, a condition that reduces your bone density and leaves you at greater risk for fractures. It is most common in menopausal and post-menopausal women but also occurs in men. There have been numerous studies that show that cardiovascular exercise, resistance training, and weight-bearing exercise can maintain—and even increase—bone mineral density. It can also assist with gait and balance, which helps to prevent falls.

Your posture is a major factor in enabling you to feel confident and attractive. It's not your individual features that count most, it's how you carry your whole body.

DO THIS

Slump your shoulders, cast your eyes downward, and drag your feet a bit. How confident do you feel when you're in that posture? Not very, right? Now straighten your spine, raise your head, and when you walk lift your feet off the ground and stride a bit. How does that feel? Pay attention to how the people around you respond to these different postures—the way you carry yourself has a huge impact!

CHAPTER 6

GET SMARTER

For years I've been telling people that exercise doesn't just do your body good, it can also make you smarter! I often hear, "Sure, Patch, but how can you *prove* that?"

Now science has proven what I've been saying all along. Thanks to brain-imaging studies in humans and neurochemical studies in animals, researchers are finding strong evidence that exercise actually helps your brain function better. Scientists have been looking closely at a protein called brain-derived neurotrophic factor (BDNF) that helps nerve cells connect in the brain. In clinical studies, rats that have BDNF levels boosted in their brains navigate mazes faster than rats whose levels hadn't been elevated. Brain injuries in high-BDNF animals also heal faster.

Scientists at Johns Hopkins University in Maryland believe that BDNF can help to rewire the brain. Even better,

they found short stints of physical activity increase BDNF
in animals' brains. In other words, *exercise* increases
BDNF! In one study, even just a *few* minutes of swimming
raised BDNF levels.

Studying BDNF in humans is more complex, but imaging techniques do show that exercise helps human brains.
Magnetic resonance imaging (MRI) has revealed that
regular exercise postpones the effects of aging in the brain.
People who exercise lose brain tissue far more slowly than
people who do not exercise. Also, exercise significantly
improves cognitive skills (such as planning and paying attention) in adults older than sixty years of age.

Physical activity that involves moderate exertion induces
cells in the brain to reinforce old connections between
neurons and to develop new connections. This greater
network of neurons means you are better able to process
and store information. In short, the more neuron connections there are in your brain, the better your brain is able
to function.

Here's the best part: you don't have to be an athlete or
run marathons to hike your IQ. Just a moderate exercise
program will boost your smarts. Every time you go for
a walk in the woods, step onto an exercise treadmill, or
swim laps in the pool, tell yourself, "I'm getting smarter!"
It's a double whammy—healthy body, healthy brain.

Did you know?

Our supersized junk-food cravings may dumb us down. Rats that were fed lots of saturated fats and sugars had significantly less BDNF (see above) in their brains than rats that were fed more nutritious food. And the adage about fish being "brain food" is true: a healthy diet high in omega-3 fatty acids such as fish oils increases BDNF in the brain. In other words, grilled salmon is going to give you more BDNF brain power than bacon.

A single piece of coconut cream pie or a cheeseburger is not going to suddenly make you dense (it might make you feel overly full and sleepy though); however, when you're preparing for an exam or an important presentation, give some thought to what you have for supper the night before.

CHOOSE FOODS WISELY

Obesity is a major health issue in our society. In fact, more than two-thirds of the North American population is overweight. When it comes to food, very often we're eating the wrong foods in the wrong proportions. We shouldn't be asking ourselves, "Did I get good value for my money—was that plate big enough to be worth the dollars spent?" Instead, we should be saying, "Did I enjoy what I ate? Does this food fuel my body? Can I trust my

body to know when it's full and not be seduced into wolf-
ing down the whole supersized serving?"

Evolution predisposed us to crave fats, which is why they
taste so good to us. Animals in the wild have a very hard
time getting fat. Have you ever seen a fat wolf or lion
(outside of the zoo, where they are passively fed)? We
humans used to be "in the wild" too. We used to have to
hunt or to gather plants for days on end. Whenever we
managed to eat some fat, it gave us a wonderful source
of long-lasting energy to keep living. That's why we love
french fries, gravy, ice cream, and other fatty foods.

But we can satisfy our centuries-old craving for fat
without reaching for junk food. There are foods that are
chock-full of healthy fats: olive, canola and flaxseed oil,
seeds, nuts, rice, and cold-water fish such as mackerel,
salmon, and tuna. In addition to the "good" fats, your
body needs fiber as well. Good fiber helps satisfy your
appetite without adding on useless calories. When you
eat fiber, make sure it's soluble. Soluble fiber absorbs and
retains water, slowing down your digestive processes. This
gives you better absorption of the nutrients in your foods,
helps to stabilize your blood sugar and lower cholesterol,
and also contributes to the health of your colon. *The top-
ten sources of soluble fiber are oats, oat bran, legumes,*

seeds, carrots, bananas, oranges, soy products, wheat bran, and rice.

Foods with antioxidant properties very often play a role in helping you maintain a healthy weight. A further benefit, however, is in how antioxidants function in our overall health. In other words, antioxidants will benefit both your waistline and your wellness.

Antioxidant foods help preserve the life of our cells and protect our hearts. Antioxidants help prevent what is called oxidative stress (damage due to oxygen), which produces free radicals (unstable molecules in our body). Free radicals are believed to be a factor in serious diseases such as Alzheimer's, ALS, diabetes, atherosclerosis, and some types of cancer. *Some great antioxidant foods are beans (kidney, pinto, and black), berries (blueberries, cranberries, raspberries, and strawberries), artichoke hearts, prunes, apples, sweet cherries, plums, and pomegranates.*

Here are some other healthy eating tips to consider. Instead of pork bacon, try turkey bacon. Instead of eating too many eggs, use egg whites (which makes for a really fluffy omelet). Instead of salt, use an herb seasoning. Instead of enriched pasta, try whole-grain pasta. Explore the world of savory herbs—rosemary, basil, thyme, mint, dill. These can add wonderful flavor to your portions and lessen your craving for excess salt.

Experiment with vegetables. Here's a recipe I made up called Citrus Stir Fry: I stir-fry vegetables along with pineapples, orange pieces, and lemon slices. You'll enjoy the really great flavor while getting vegetables and fruit in the same entrée!

The combination of good nutrition, regular exercise, and portion control of your food will go a long way to helping you achieve an energetic healthy life and a good weight.

DO THIS:

This week, include some well-known brain foods in your meals. Whenever possible, eat fresh vegetables rather than frozen or canned. And don't forget to drink approximately eight eight-ounce glasses of water per day. However, also realize that your water needs can vary according to your weight and lifestyle. The 'eight by eight' rule is a general recommendation only. If you have questions about your specific water intake, it's a good idea to check with your doctor.

CHAPTER 7

BURN OFF YOUR BURNOUT

These days we must manage multiple levels of stress at once. As a result, burnout is reaching epidemic proportions. Perhaps you're a single parent who works a demanding job and also cares for your aging parents; or maybe you're an entrepreneur dealing with the stress of growing your company. Or maybe you're coping with a chronic condition such as diabetes or arthritis. The world continues to get more competitive and stressful, and sometimes you get to the point where you say, "I'm at the end of my rope."

This is often the moment you want to crash in front of the TV. But guess what? Being a couch potato will only *increase* your feelings of exhaustion. One of the culprits is cortisol, often called the "stress hormone." To maintain a normal metabolism, your body needs to produce a certain level of cortisol. But high levels of stress—the feeling of having too much on our plate and not enough time in a day—cause our cortisol levels to fluctuate wildly, making us feel "wired": tired, with stiff muscles, yet unable to relax. You know the kind of feeling I'm talking about—when your nerves feel like guitar strings about to snap. If your cortisol levels are chronically elevated, this will have a negative effect on your sleep, your mood, your sex drive, your bones and ligaments, plus your heart and lungs. So "relaxing" in front of the TV is not enough.

Did you know?

The average North American watches television an estimated twenty to twenty-eight hours a week.

Physical exercise helps to normalize cortisol levels and to prevent irregular fluctuations of this complex hormone. It also modulates your body's production of adrenaline (which in too high amounts also contributes to feeling "wired"), turning it into noradrenalin, which is more calming to the body and so improves your body's ability to deal with stress. So, in the same way that you think about exercise as burning off calories, think of yourself as burning off stress. *You are literally burning off the stressed-out feeling that made you feel run-down in the first place.* Five hours of passively staring at a TV screen won't do that for you, but *twenty minutes* of exercise will!

With a renewed sense of energy, take an inventory of your life. Consider which parts of your life you need to change. What things you might be doing that drain your energy that you could let go of. If you're a stressed-out manager, learn to delegate. Come up with a way to share chores more equitably at home. Take that vacation you've been putting off. And, of course, even just a little exercise will help you cope and you'll feel better quickly!

If you allow your body to naturally get its mojo back through physical activity, the "burn" you feel will be transformed into a "flame" ... your zest for living.

Did you know?

American health psychologist and leadership writer Dr. Robert K. Cooper writes in his book, *The Other 90%*, that human beings use only 10 percent or less of their true potential. One of the ways Cooper suggests accessing "the other 90 percent" is through cultivating calm energy. His recommendations include becoming aware of your posture (finding the body's natural stance); deep-breathing patterns; enjoying physical activity; and relaxing your mind—all of which are the goals of a good fitness program.

INVEST IN A LITTLE "ME TIME"

A lot of parents feel guilty about leaving their kids and going to the gym. Instead of giving yourself a hard time, consider your workouts a benefit to your family. Giving yourself a little "me time" every day enables you to take care of yourself, gain energy, and be there for others. It sets a great lifetime example for your children. In many fitness clubs you will find child-minding areas because we know that giving moms and dads an opportunity to work out gives them renewed energy to deal with the many demands of parenthood.

DO THIS

This week, list the top-five "burnouts" in your life. Now list five activities that could lift you out of the burnout. Make sure to put exercise *high* on your list. Other options could include:

- Delegate or share tasks at work if possible. Take pride in the work you do.
- Work out a schedule for sharing household chores. (In other words, don't do them all yourself!) Post a list on the fridge or some other prominent location, inviting every member of your household to complete three chores of their choice.
- Take up a new hobby—such as yoga, woodworking, or volunteering.
- Get back in touch. Call up someone you've wanted to see and go out for coffee, lunch, or a walk.
- See what is *right* with your life and make *that* the focus of your thoughts.
- Believe that by taking responsibility you have the power to make changes.

CHAPTER 8

A NATURAL TREATMENT FOR DEPRESSION

Depression is the most prevalent mental health problem in North America, yet it is often undiagnosed or under-diagnosed, leaving vast numbers of people suffering in silence. Did you know that one of the best treatments for depression is exercise?

There is a neurochemical basis for depression. Many clinically depressed people have low levels of a brain chemical called serotonin. Low serotonin is associated with anxiety, racing thoughts, chronic pain, and altered sleep patterns—all symptoms of depression. There are some powerful physiological and psychological reasons exercise can help with depression.

First, physical movement helps elevate the level of serotonin in your brain, and when your serotonin levels are raised, you experience a sense of confidence and well-being.

Second, you experience a boost in your self-esteem by taking an active role in your own recovery. Exercising is not passive. Some forms of exercise, such as group exercise classes, personal training in a group, playing on a recreational sports team, joining a walking club, taking a yoga class, or playing pick-up hockey, help create connections with others, which can also boost your mood.

Third, the pleasant mood induced by your endorphins released during exercise may help to break the cycle of pessimistic thinking—if you feel good, you are less likely to feel overwhelmed by negative thoughts.

I can tell you that after thirty years of watching people in my fitness clubs, one of the greatest benefits of exercise is the feeling of self-control it provides. You might not be able to control your boss and co-workers, family, or politicians, bankers, and the tax department. You can, however, control your physical activity. You can see exercise as a key step in taking control of your life. With exercise, you can think more clearly and control your waistline, attitude, health, and self-awareness.

THE RESULTS ARE IN
In *SPARK*, a book on the science of exercise and the brain, Harvard professor and psychiatrist Dr. James Ratey writes about a study that examined the effects of exercise

and drug therapy in treating depression. The study involved 156 depressed men and women. The patients were divided into three groups. Over sixteen weeks one group took antidepressants, the second group did an aerobic exercise program, and the third group used both medication and exercise. The result? All three groups showed a significant decrease in depression, and about half of each group was, to quote Ratey, "completely out of the woods—in remission."

Did you know?

If you exercise, you may not need to take as much antidepressant medication. Because exercise can improve your serotonin levels, it may be possible to manage on a lower dose of medication. There is evidence also that treatment for depression, *if accompanied by exercise*, can lead to a faster recovery time. If you are being treated for depression, always talk to your doctor before considering lowering your medication. Your doctor can work with you to create a treatment plan that is right for you.

To add further to the intriguing possibilities of exercise, Dr. Ratey reports that a study of thirty depressed patients "showed that every one of them had lower than normal

BDNF levels." (Remember that BDNF is the protein in your brain that boosts your brain's ability to function.) In another study, "antidepressants restored depressed patients' BDNF levels to normal, and yet another showed that higher levels of BDNF correspond to fewer symptoms." In other words, it appears that BDNF can be affected by depression and that it too plays a role in how we feel. It's not uncommon for depressed individuals to say that they feel they're in a "brain fog" and that their mind just won't work the way it used to. It's possible that the link between depression and BDNF levels could help explain why.

In an animal model, Ratey reports that "exercise boosts BDNF at least as much as antidepressants, and sometimes more.... And in humans we know that exercise raises BDNF, at least in the bloodstream, much like antidepressants do."

DO THIS

If you are suffering from depression, team up with your doctor to explore all the treatment options. Make sure that your doctor includes exercise. The only side effects of exercise are positive ones. Through exercise, you can become a participant in your own health care and an active partner in breaking the cycle of depression. You can reclaim your energy and your life.

CHAPTER 9

KEEP YOUR BRAIN ON EXERCISE

Computer programs aimed at improving your brain's performance—games such as Sudoku (a complicated game of numbers and squares) or Dragger (involving dragging and dropping pieces of an image to form a whole picture, a type of cyber jigsaw puzzle, so to speak)—are a booming industry today. In the United States, consumers are predicted to spend more than $80 million a year on brain exercise products, a considerable increase from $2 million in 2005. One thing about "brain games"—they are a fantastic alternative to watching TV.

It's certainly true that a stimulating environment improves our ability to function. When animals used in laboratory experiments, such as rats or monkeys, are given toys or playmates, they learn to handle a multitude of tasks very easily. We've certainly seen that children thrive in stimulating settings with vibrant colors and lots of things to do.

When we're bored, we feel less energetic. When our interest is captivated, we feel alive.

Having a stimulating hobby, setting new goals at work, or learning a new language all have positive effects on our mental health and on our mind's ability to function. However, I don't think we should trick ourselves into believing that doing "brain exercises" on a computer or pursuing a hobby or goal *alone* will help guard our total mental function.

The bottom line is that physical exercise is one of the best ways to keep your mind intact. It increases the number of connections between the neurons, and it slows down the inevitable age-related shrinking of the frontal cortex of your brain (associated with attention, long-term memory, and planning). Exercise also increases the capillaries in your brain, leading to better blood flow, and it improves your cardiovascular health, which helps prevent heart attacks and strokes that can cause brain damage.

I'm not telling you to give up your hobbies, or to stop doing puzzles or other brain-teasing activities—these do play a role in keeping your brain up to speed. Instead, I'm asking you to add physical activity to the mix!

Did you know?

There is evidence that a physical activity as simple as walking helps protect you from developing dementia in your senior years. A four-year study reported in the December 2007 issue of *The Journal of Neurology* involving 749 women and men older than sixty-five years of age found that the top one-third of people who exerted the most energy walking (by pumping their arms or walking at a fast pace) were 27 percent less likely to develop vascular dementia than those in the bottom third. People who used the most energy in moderate physical activity were 29 percent less likely to develop the condition, and those in the top one-third for total physical activity had an overall 24 percent reduced risk of developing dementia compared to the bottom third.

EXERCISE BOOSTS YOUR JOB PERFORMANCE

Some research from the United Kingdom has given strong support to the idea that busy workers who exercise during the day are more productive and less likely to be irritable with colleagues. The researchers studied two hundred workers in three different job environments: a university, a computer company, and a life insurance company. Employees filled out questionnaires about their job performance and their mood on days when they exercised at work and on days when they didn't.

The participants were free to choose the physical activity. The majority spent thirty to sixty minutes during their lunch break doing group exercise, strength training, yoga, and/or playing pick-up basketball games.

Two-thirds of the employees found that their time-management skills, mental performance, and ability to meet deadlines improved on the days when they exercised. The overall boost to better performance was an impressive 15 percent.

The interesting thing was that the *type* of exercise didn't matter. The same performance-boosting effect resulted from a simple brisk walk as from more elaborate sports-related activities. The important thing was to get the body moving.

The employees also rated their moods in the morning and afternoon. The overwhelming majority of employees reported that exercise put them "in a good mood." During focus group discussions, many said they experienced a more accepting attitude toward themselves and their work and were better able to take their work challenges in stride. They didn't lose their temper as much and found that episodes of irritability were significantly reduced. They also reported that they were not experiencing feelings of fatigue in the afternoon. Herein lies exercise's wonderful paradox—that by expending energy, you get more energy in return.

DO THIS

Instead of simply solving puzzles in a book or playing games on the computer, go to the fitness club *first* and get your body moving, *then* enjoy your brain teasers. Did you do better after your workout?

CHAPTER 10

HEART HEALTH

If you or someone you love has heart disease, forgoing exercise may be the worst thing you can do. Research shows that exercise actually helps your body create new blood vessels, both around your heart and throughout your body. These blood vessels carry the oxygen and nutrients all over your body. These nutrients are necessary for life.

A 2007 study headed by Dr. Robert Hollriegel at Leipzig University in Germany found that people with serious heart problems who rode a bicycle for up to half an hour each day produced more stem cells in their bones and were found to have more small blood vessels in their muscles than patients who didn't exercise. (They had no change in their blood vessels or muscles.)

What does this mean? Physical activity causes a tenfold increase in blood sent to the muscles, which puts a "strain" on the heart's arteries and muscles. In response to this, your body sends stem cells to the site of the stress. The stem cells are believed to play a role in repairing the damage. The researchers hypothesized that if you're a heart patient and you continue to exercise, this could create even more stem cells to help your heart recover or, at the very least, to improve. The formation of new blood vessels and the increased strength in the muscles as a result of exercise may also help with rehabilitating the heart. This only happens, though, if you continue to exercise *regularly.*

Even though the study was looking at heart patients, we shouldn't miss the message about prevention: *exercise is a lifesaver.* It reduces your risk of heart disease and stroke—and improves your odds of recovering. Lack of exercise makes it more difficult for your heart to function well, which leaves you feeling short of breath. Then you become afraid to exercise. It's a vicious cycle! The key to overcoming this fear is to talk to your doctor about how to gradually include exercise in your day-to-day life and then start out slowly.

Don't expect to do the exercises perfectly; just do what you can handle and gradually do a little more week by week, under your doctor's supervision. Soon you'll lose the fear as you begin to feel the benefits of exercise. The day will come when you notice that you aren't as out of breath as before and that you have more energy. Take it one step at a time.

Medical associations recommend exercise, and many doctors now prescribe physical activity as a matter of course. Perhaps it's time that all doctors write prescriptions for exercise the same way they write prescriptions for medications!

PREVENTION OF HEART DISEASE:
RISK FACTORS YOU CAN HELP CONTROL

1. **Being overweight:** Almost two-thirds of North Americans are overweight. Achieving and maintaining a healthy weight can help prevent heart attacks.

2. **High blood pressure:** Many adults don't realize they have high blood pressure because it often has no symptoms, yet it is one of the vmajor risk factors in heart attacks. Check your blood pressure regularly, and don't forget that regular exercise helps keep blood pressure within a healthy range.

3. **High blood cholesterol:** Cholesterol is a type of fat in your blood. Good cholesterol, called high density lipoprotein (HDL), helps take the "bad" cholesterol away from artery walls. The "bad" cholesterol, or low density lipoprotein (LDL), adheres to your artery walls and causes plaque to build up. Reduce your fat intake to 20 percent to 35 percent of your daily food. Get physical. Exercise can help lower the bad cholesterol.

4. **Physical inactivity**: *If you're physically inactive, you have twice the risk for heart disease.* Half-hour periods of exercise several times a week should become part of your heart health lifestyle.

5. **Excessive consumption of alcohol**: Very moderate use of alcohol such as red wine may help your heart. However, drinking *too much* of any kind of alcohol can increase your blood pressure and contribute to heart risk factors.

6. **Smoking**: We all know smoking's terrible effect on the lungs. Its effect on the heart is just as lethal. Smoking increases your risk of blood clots, reduces the oxygen in your blood, increases the plaque in your arteries, and makes your heart work a lot harder. Bluntly put, you will die a lot sooner if you smoke.

7. **Diabetes**: Regular exercise can help prevent type 2 diabetes. If you do have diabetes, learn about healthy eating from a professional dietician, achieve and maintain a healthy weight, and exercise.

8. **Stress**: Too much stress can increase risk for your heart.

DO THIS

Put your whole heart into exercise! For the next ten minutes, write down all the reasons you exercise (or want to start). Even if you end up repeating some of your reasons, don't stop writing! When the ten minutes are up, read all your reasons and put them into categories. These might be losing weight, improving your appearance, living longer, improving your quality of life, or even just for the sheer pleasure of it! For example, if you wrote, "Keeping my blood sugar under control," your reason falls under Living Longer. If you wrote, "I want to play with my kids or grandkids without getting winded," your reason falls under Quality of Life, and so forth.

Now pick one key reason from each category and think of a physical activity that can help get you that result. This coming week, commit yourself to doing at least one, and preferably two, of the activities you've chosen. In this way, you are bringing consciousness to the way you exercise. You're showing up in your own life.

PART II

EXERCISE, TAKE THE FIRST STEP

A few years ago, I was giving a speech at a high school in my home province of Ontario. The physical education teacher had posted a large sign in the gym that read, "You must show up to win." The sign didn't guarantee that students would automatically win every game they ever played. It implied that the first step toward the *possibility* of winning was in showing up. It's the same with your life: Show up in your own life—and to your exercise routine—and you'll be giving yourself the chance to win at life in more ways than you could ever imagine.

In Part I, I talked a lot about *why* you should exercise—all the great things physical activity can do for you. In Part II, we're going to delve into a bit of the psychology around exercise, particularly looking at the thoughts and feelings that might prevent you from getting physical. For example, you may be thinking:

"People are looking at me!"

"Have I started too late? Am I too old?"

"Will I have the time?"

We'll also be talking about your body type and how each body type responds to exercise. And we'll have some fun with how you become an "attractor" (the physical reasons behind that) and how laughter is not only the best medicine, it's exercise too! My hope is that after reading Part II, you'll have plenty of motivation to stay in the right mental space to be successful with your exercise program.

People often ask me, "What keeps you motivated? How do you get up at 6 a.m. for a workout? How do you work out at night? Won't you be too tired after all those hours of work? Won't it interfere with your sleep?"

The answer to staying motivated is twofold. First, avoid all the pain that accompanies not exercising by instead … you guessed it … exercising. Second, give yourself rewards. Many of us have an inner script that plays on repeat inside our heads: "Oh, life can be such a drag. I'm tired. I'm no good at exercise. I'm too stressed out." These are all negative messages—you're making yourself feel bad, which never motivated anyone to do anything! This applies to everything you do in your life. No one achieves a dream or a goal by continually reciting all the things that might stop them from getting there.

Instead, play with all the different ways you can incorporate positive messages into your thinking and into your life. Begin each day by smiling at yourself in the mirror. Compliment yourself for getting out of bed. Remind yourself how good a hot shower feels. Eat something nutritious for breakfast.

Before you get started, please don't get caught up in the "perfect image" media hype or the myth of the "perfect exerciser." Those images have nothing to do with real life. If you buy into them, you'll drive yourself crazy and quit.

It's also important not to berate yourself if you occasionally skip your exercise. Instead, make the decision to return to it the next day, and when you get there, compliment yourself for getting back on track. This isn't about perfection, it's about being the best you that you can be. There's nothing egotistical about complimenting yourself. There's nothing self-absorbed about noticing your little victories each day, no matter how small they may seem. Everything in life comes down to one step at a time.

People in my clubs frequently share their stories with me, and often they really move me. One of my club members, Krista, told me how she made the decision to show up in her own life and be the best she could be, despite significant medical setbacks. Krista's story is inspirational on two fronts. First, she is an example of giving her all in the face of obstacles. And second, it's about learning the wisdom of "good enough is good enough"—that you don't have to be perfect.

Krista had been physically active since high school. When she was twenty-six, she slipped on a grassy hill and hurt her ankle. She didn't think anything of it—ankle sprains are fairly common and usually heal pretty quickly. But Krista noticed that her ankle didn't seem to be recovering well and decided to get a referral to a physiotherapist. The physiotherapist tested Krista's reflexes. With a concerned look on her face, the physiotherapist told Krista that a physical response known as hyper-reflexia was present, which can indicate severe upper-neurological damage, often the result of a stroke or past trauma.

Krista immediately thought of the severe car accident she had been in a few years prior. Emergency department doctors at the time had initially suspected that Krista had broken her neck but eventually gave her the all-clear.

Now, several years later, Krista began a difficult journey through the health-care system. At first the neurologists thought it was a brain tumor, or perhaps multiple sclerosis (MS), but both were ruled out. They finally diagnosed Krista with a condition known as Arnold-Chiari malformation, which she, like most of us, had never heard of.

Her cerebellum was growing into her neck and, as a result, nerves were being crushed in her spinal column. The neurologists told her that the condition had likely been present since birth but was only manifesting now. Magnetic resonance imaging (MRI) also revealed a lesion in her spinal column, which one neurosurgeon thought was MS, but the neurologist disagreed. There was no consensus about the cause of the lesion. The medical team decided to perform brain surgery to fix the malformation and hoped that the lesion would resolve itself on its own.

Throughout it all, Krista kept working out. But as the time for her surgery drew near, she realized that her right side was weaker than her left and that she was no longer able to run. Walking was also becoming a challenge. The surgeon repaired the malformation and told her that she wouldn't deteriorate further, but that her present condition would be the "new normal" and that she might as well just get used to it.

She was shocked. Krista asked for a referral to physio-
therapy and was anxious to return to exercise, since she
felt that exercise would play a huge role in her recovery.
She figured that if stroke patients can relearn to walk and
talk, she, too, could rebuild her weakened body. Even
when the neurologist told her that the spinal lesion was
still there and that MS was still "on the table," Krista
refused to be discouraged.

She began going to her local GoodLife fitness club, where
the staff was encouraging and worked with her to help
her make gains at her own pace. Krista says:

> On the days that were really hard—when my neck
> pain was almost debilitating and my workouts
> weren't very good, or I tripped and fell off the
> treadmill, scraping my knees—I always remembered
> Patch's words: "Good enough is good enough."
> What a brilliant concept! I would give it my best
> each day and that was good enough!

> I spent the next two years having MRIs and spinal
> taps and at the end of the day I am still a medical
> mystery … I had two rare, unrelated neurological
> disorders. When put together they dramatically com-
> promised my motor control and balance. I didn't

have MS, but no one figured out what the mystery spot on my spinal cord was.

I was still able to walk and talk and go to the gym every day. I couldn't do everything I had in the past, but I had discovered that I could experience fitness in a whole new way. Even with my limitations, I could still feel good and get my body to perform better than it would if I didn't exercise. I am a lot healthier than I would be if it were not for my workouts.

I am a success story. I still trip and fall a few times a day, but I am okay. I have found a new way to appreciate fitness in my life. With the help of the fitness staff at the club, I have modified what I do. I reframed my training into what I *can* accomplish, not what I am unable to do. For that I will be forever thankful.

For Krista, "one step at a time" took on poignant meaning. She stopped focusing on her former athletic "perfection" and instead used exercise as a way to keep showing up in her own life. Many of us do not have the challenges Krista has, but we can all learn something from her attitude. Even with serious physical challenges it is possible to say "yes" to physical activity. We can take hope from this. Our own efforts to give ourselves the gift of exercise will increase our sense of self-control, self-esteem, and confidence. This is what I want for you.

All I'm asking of you is to commit to regular physical activity. Thirty minutes, three times a week. Imagine— thirty minutes to achieve the real sexy, smart, and strong. You really can do this! If you can show up for exercise for a total of ninety minutes over a week's time, you will change your life for the better.

CHAPTER 11

THE STAGES OF EXERCISE: WHAT TO EXPECT

It's important to understand that there are primarily three stages to becoming fit. Many people quit exercising too early on in the process because they don't realize that just halting the process of physical decline is a major accomplishment. They may set goals for themselves that are unrealistic. Or they keep setting goals that are more and more challenging when instead they should be saying, "I'm okay right now." If you know that there are three stages, your mind can work with you to help you stay on course.

The first exciting stage is that you stop getting worse. In other words, you stop putting on weight (or put it on at a slower rate) and you stop getting weaker, which is a major victory in itself. Recognize that you've taken a major step toward making yourself better. Don't scold yourself about the distance you have yet to cover. Instead, use your mind to reinforce the fact that you have achieved step one.

In the second wondrous stage, you begin to reverse damage. Let's say you're fifty pounds (twenty-three kilograms) overweight and you set an interim goal of losing twenty pounds (nine kilograms). When you get to that point, celebrate! Sure, you still have thirty pounds (fourteen kilograms) to go, but by tackling the initial twenty, you've already won! Be proud of yourself for getting this far—it will help you stay motivated to drop the next thirty pounds and arrive at your ideal weight and fitness level.

The third and most satisfying stage is about maintenance—where you reach your own personal goals of equilibrium and optimum health and you work to stay at that level. It's like brushing your teeth—it's the difference between keeping your teeth or not. Just keep doing the same workout year in and year out. Victory! Good enough is good enough.

There is no magic lottery that will give you a healthy body and sharp mind. But you *can* win the game with "good enough is good enough." Your body is wonderful. It doesn't need perfection. It just needs a level where it works well and you feel good.

Did you know?

Slow steady progress is much more effective and will likely make it easier for you to maintain your health than rapid progress. When things happen too fast, you can get into the "yo-yo syndrome" of losing momentum and slipping back, then trying again (which can quickly become self-defeating). As they say in the tale of the tortoise and the hare—"Slow and steady wins the race."

THE OPTIONAL FOURTH STAGE

There is a place for what I call a fourth stage of fitness. Less than 2 percent of the population is interested in the fourth stage, which is the achievement of *maximum* fitness levels. Unless you're an elite athlete or have a short-term goal such as running a marathon by the time you're forty, you don't need maximum fitness levels.

That said, if you do want to feel the rush—the challenge and the purpose of doing something physical to the best of your ability, even if it's only a one-time thing—then go for it! It's totally worth the effort. A great example of this is my good friend Jane, who in her late forties ran the Midnight Sun Marathon in Arctic Bay, Nunavut, in Canada's Arctic region. Jane trained hard for four months, running ten to twenty-two miles (sixteen to thirty-five kilometers) on a weekend, and doing shorter runs during the week, as well as core strength training. On top of the physical benefit of giving yourself a challenge such as this, you grow in self-respect, competitiveness, discipline, and intelligence. You will heighten your awareness, your optimism, and your ability to persevere.

As I've mentioned, it's not necessary for you to go to this fourth stage. It's entirely your choice. Just taking yourself through the three stages is more than enough. However, if you're an individual who really wants a big physical challenge, then you *might* choose to give yourself a fourth-stage experience.

DO THIS

If you're just starting to exercise after a period of inactivity, get a journal and start by writing "Stage One: The Buck Stops Here." Each day, jot down what you did that was physical. In the margins, write, "The buck stops here. I'm ready to be in better health."

When you start to see some results—when you've lost five pounds (two kilograms) or gained a bit of muscle—add this heading: "Stage Two: Reversing the Damage." Keep jotting down what physical things you did, and in the margins write, "I am moving toward better health, more happiness, and boundless energy."

When you reach your fitness goal, add the heading "Stage Three: Good Enough Is Good Enough." Continue to record your physical activities in a small diary entry, and in the margin write, "I'm good, life is good, my body's good, all of me is good … good enough is good enough!"

CHAPTER 12

NO MATTER WHAT YOUR BODY TYPE

Before you get started, keep this in mind: each person has a different body type—scientists call this your somatotype. One of the reasons that many people feel unhappy with their bodies is that they are fixated on achieving a look that is outside the realm of their particular body type. This is an exercise in futility. I don't want you exercising for futility; I want you exercising for *results*.

You'll find that if you go *with* your body type, you'll get the best results for *you*. There are three main body types: ectomorph, endomorph, and mesomorph.

An ectomorph is naturally slender. He or she has long limbs, a slender trunk, a smaller chest frame, hip girdle, and bones, and narrow shoulders. This is my body type. Some well-known examples of this body type are actors Jim Carrey and Gwyneth Paltrow.

An endomorph has a rounder physique. If you're an endomorph, you have rounder thighs and arms and a fuller face and chest. Think of singer Jennifer Hudson and comedian Robin Williams.

The mesomorph has a more muscular frame, smaller hips, and larger shoulders. Sometimes these types seem to be muscular without doing anything. Examples of this body type are golfer Tiger Woods and actor Halle Berry.

Everyone is a combination of these different types, but one type usually dominates. With exercise, the ectomorph will gain muscle and become stronger. The endomorph will lose some of the roundness and put on some muscle. The mesomorph will become more dramatically muscular.

Did you know?

Nature equipped male and female bodies with different evolutionary traits. In prehistoric times, females tended to be the gatherers. They were the child-bearers and thus evolved to have more substantial hips, making their center of gravity lower. Women carry fat first and foremost on their derrieres and thighs. This keeps their body fat out of the way of bending and picking up objects and children. For the most part, men were the hunters (of course there were female hunters, but the majority of prehistoric hunting was done by men). As a result, men needed to run, either toward or away from something. So the best place to store fat was in their abdomen, where it would help protect their inner organs and not slow down their legs if an animal charged. We still carry these evolutionary patterns, courtesy of Mother Nature. So if you're working on losing weight, remember this: the last place women will typically lose weight will be on their hips and derriere, and men will lose their belly fat last.

Each type tends to excel at different types of sports—endomorphs and mesomorphs may be great swimmers because they have more body fat to support them in the water. The long linear ectomorph does better on *top* of the water—as rowers, for example. (Rowing has been my particular competitive sport.) But unless you want to be an Olympic athlete, this type of body classification is not all that useful for your favorite sport (although it *is* useful for your fitness program). Elite athletes do have to consider whether their body type is suitable for their sport, and you have to consider your body type in terms of your exercise results in the sense that if you're hoping to become a first-class athlete, your body type needs to be right for the sport. If you're just doing a sport for recreation, not for high-end competition, don't worry about your body type. Just do what you enjoy.

For example, in marathon running the elite male runners are ideally 135 pounds (61 kilograms), slim, and around five-foot-five (165 centimeters). Yet millions of people of all shapes and sizes run marathons, not for the medals but for the sheer accomplishment of just doing it. I ran the Boston Marathon at 225 pounds (102 kilograms) and I'm six-foot-four (193 centimeters). Did I finish first or in the top ten? No way! Did I finish the race itself? Yes, and that was enough for me!

Basically, taking your body type into account when you create your personal exercise program is about setting your future sights correctly, loving yourself and your beauty as they are, and enjoying new feelings of health and vitality in your body. Consider that you are doing it to improve the body you already have. Don't stress yourself out trying to be something you're not. As an ectomorph, there's no way that I'm going to achieve the compact muscular chest of the mesomorph, and there's no way an endomorph is suddenly going to grow several inches to become an ectomorph. The good news is that all three of these body types look terrific when their body is healthy, full of energy, and fit.

DO THIS

Stand in front of a mirror and identify your natural body type. See if you can tell whether you're an ectomorph, endomorph, or mesomorph. If you seem to have characteristics of two or all three, try to determine which type predominates. Set a goal to make your body the best it can be, according to your type, not someone else's. Each of these three body types can be vibrant, sexy, and strong.

CHAPTER 13

WHO'S LOOKING?

Throughout my career in the fitness business, I've became aware of one major obstacle that prevents people from really getting into their bodies: the fear of being looked at. It can stop people from putting some *oomph* into exercise.

Because we are taught to be hyper-aware of our physical imperfections, we tend to exaggerate how much everyone else notices them too. Many times people have said to me, "Patch, I'm just so self-conscious about exercising. I see all those people who are such good shape, and I can't help but compare myself to them. I don't want people watching me!"

I understand this feeling, since I had to come to terms with it myself. I'm a normal guy, but because of my tall height I used to worry that I would be readily noticeable and that everyone would know if I did something wrong during my exercise routine. I'd think, "Everyone's going to be watching me. After all, I'm the owner of this club! People are going to expect me to have perfect form when I strength train or do a stretch class." I'd feel particularly self-conscious when I'd have a rheumatoid arthritis flare-up, leaving me temporarily weak and feeble.

Well, it wasn't long before I realized the truth: *no one was looking at me!* Most people didn't even know I existed. And those who did usually glanced over, smiled, engaged me in a bit of conversation, but then got right back to their own workout. For the most part, people were absorbed in what *they* were doing—listening to their music or just enjoying being in the zone working out.

When you can exercise with the consciousness that no one is going to notice your less-than-perfect maneuvers (other than your fitness instructor or personal trainer, whose job it is to notice!), you give yourself the inner freedom to focus on how good you feel. You can relax and just be yourself.

This is true not just for exercising in fitness clubs or playing a sport. It can apply to being on the beach or at a party. As you get more comfortable in your own skin, you can relax into your own physical being. Then a paradoxical thing happens: people *do* start looking at you! They're being attracted to your energy. People who are comfortable with themselves make others feel at ease and, as a result, draw people to them.

YOU LIKE *WHAT* ABOUT ME?

How often have you focused on one of your so-called flaws only to have someone compliment you on that very thing? Let's say you've got really curly hair, but you've always wished you had straight hair. Then you meet someone who says, "I just love your curly hair!" Perhaps you're in a group fitness class and you don't think you've got the rhythm quite right, and the person next to you says, "You're so good at that! Can I stand next to you in the next class too?"

Take a moment to ask yourself what you get complimented on. When I present a seminar or workshop at fitness organizations around the world, I ask people to get into small groups and talk about what they admire about one another. People often gain new insights into themselves. Sometimes people say, "I didn't think that I had that great a laugh, but she seems to really appreciate it." Or "I've always seen myself as shy and reserved, but someone in the group just told me that I seem thoughtful and reflective."

It's impossible to predict exactly what about us draws other people in, so there's no point worrying about it!

DO THIS

The next time you want to compliment someone, don't keep it to yourself. Say it to them!

CHAPTER 14

MAKING "SCENTS" OF HOW YOU ATTRACT

Here's something to think about as you learn to show up in your own life and take some chances on becoming the real sexy, smart, and strong that you are. Why do we find one person attractive and not another? Maybe the person in your fitness class is the best-looking person you've seen in a long time, but they just don't do anything for you. Maybe the person seated next to you in the theater isn't exactly a rival for your favorite movie star, yet there's something about him or her that makes you want to strike up a conversation. Chances are some of that un-explainable attraction comes down to your sense of smell. I don't mean perfume or aftershave. I mean the smells you can't even detect—the ones emanating from the hormonal mixture in our bodies.

The actual chemistry of sexual attractiveness is quite complex. It has to do with hormones such as estrogen and testosterone, brain chemicals such as dopamine, and the pheromones found in our body sweat. Indeed, scent and the sense of smell may be the overall number-one predictor of physical sexual attraction, according to scientists who study the complexities of what creates sexual desire.

Did you know?

Many animals in the wild can smell a potential mate from quite a distance. Even domestic dogs and cats have this keen sense of smell. We humans do still have a sense of smell, but it's nowhere near as sensitive as that of our four-legged friends. We've become so addicted to masking our natural body scent with perfumes and aftershave that our sense of smell, in terms of detecting pheromones, has become weaker.

Romance experts often advise us to cut back on perfume or aftershave, or to wear just a dash, so as not to compete so much with our natural pheromones. Sure, people wearing perfume and aftershave do get together—that's Mother Nature's ingenuity. Despite all the decidedly non-human scents we put onto our skin, those persistent pheromones can still sneak through—our scented products just make it harder to do. You may be even more attractive (pheromonically speaking) if you don't wear perfumes and instead just go with the natural scent of your body. This doesn't mean that you shouldn't shower or that you should rush home all sweaty from the gym expecting your partner to think, "How wonderful!"

One of the benefits of knowing about hormones and pheromones is that they contribute to the mating game and they happen naturally. Attraction, on the physical level at least, partially depends on whether someone's pheromones pick up yours. Usually our pheromones cause us to feel attracted to someone whose genetic makeup is different from our own. This is one of nature's ways of ensuring successful reproduction. Since detecting pheromones is below our conscious threshold (in other words, we smell them, but we don't know we're smelling them), there's no point in worrying. You just can't know. It's the luck of the draw!

Knowing this can free you up to concentrate on making your body as vital and healthy as possible. You can't control whether somebody is going to "dig" you from across a crowded room, but you *can* control how you feel when you're in that room. If you've got that inner glow of health, those shining eyes, and the comfort level with your own body that you get with regular exercise, believe me, someone is going to detect your pheromones!

BEYOND THE PHEROMONES ...

The chemistry of the body is *not* the only thing that draws us to others. Other qualities play a big role. This was really brought home to me by a recent survey we did at my GoodLife clubs, with more than 3,000 of our members responding. As part of the research for this book, we sent out a questionnaire asking, "What do you find attractive in a person?" Overwhelmingly, the major qualities people named were a positive attitude, a confident bearing, a great smile, a sense of humor, and the idea that people who appear to take care of themselves are attractive.

- 72 percent said that feeling at home in their body boosts their self-esteem.
- 66 percent said they felt it's important to maintain their sense of attractiveness as they age.
- More than 50 percent said that physical activity was a major factor in why they felt comfortable.

They rated the actual exercise components themselves over healthy eating and stress reduction—both of which are other major reasons for joining a fitness club. It's interesting that most members found that *doing* the physical activity, not necessarily the results, is the most important aspect of feeling good about themselves.

Here are some wonderful comments from the survey:

- "I feel sexiest when I am able to push myself past my comfort zone, either mentally or physically."
- "I believe that sexy is a state of mind and in order to feel positive, you need to perform positive actions—eat well, exercise, get the most out of life."
- "I feel very fit for my age and I think that makes me feel sexy. I'm in better shape at age fifty than I was at twenty-five, or even eighteen for that matter!"

DO THIS

Switch to unscented soap and hair products and try forgoing perfume or scented aftershave for a period of time. Put some trust in your pheromones to do some attracting for you, and meanwhile *you* work on your fitness so that your body always feels great.

CHAPTER 15

YOU'VE BEEN WORKING OUT, HAVEN'T YOU?

Members of my clubs often joke about my "sixth sense." "Hey, Patch," they say, "I bet you can tell when you walk into a room full of strangers who works out and who doesn't! I bet you have a fitness radar." Well, actually, I do. Perhaps because I've spent most of my life being passionate about fitness, health, and well-being, I have trained my eyes and ears to be alert for the fitness signals (or non-fitness signals) emanating from people.

If I were to meet you at a conference or at the supermarket, how would I know if you exercise? People who work out tend to have lots of energy. You can see the bounce in their step. They hold their bodies in a strong, upright posture and there is purposefulness in their stride. They smile a lot and their eyes are clear and alert. They're not out of breath or wheezing. Even if they do not yet have the weight level they are aiming for, their skin has a healthy glow and you can feel their optimism about life.

The fit person is the one in the room at the end of a long day who is not spent. He or she can be in the middle of chaos and not get fazed. Fit people don't have any problems bending or stretching, so if I see a person bend down to pick a heavy box, for example, I'll know from the way he holds his body whether he's an exerciser. If I see a person take the stairs quickly and lightly, I'll know she likely works out.

Body language tells me a lot about where people are at with exercise. If I were to meet you tomorrow, what would I see about you? More importantly, how do you want people to see you?

DO THIS

The next time you are on the subway, at a baseball game or a dance, observe various people's body language. Look at their posture, their energy, the way they move. See if you can intuitively tell who might exercise regularly. Then, if you have a chance to strike up a conversation, say, "You seem to be in really good shape. You've got so much energy." Chances are they'll tell you that they play a sport, belong to a fitness club, or love to walk, skate, or ski.

CHAPTER 16

TOO BUSY TO EXERCISE?

A lot of people just don't know how to fit exercise into their schedules. Maybe you're a single parent, a busy executive, or a stressed-out college student. We often feel like we don't have the time to add exercise to the mix. But the truth is, with some planning and imagination, you can always make the time.

If you're a parent, choose a club that has child care or arrange to have your partner make dinner so that you can go out for a pre-dinner run, to the club, or a walk. If you have a small child, exercise at home using rubber tubing or a balance ball while your baby has a nap. If you're a student, you could go to the gym on your campus as a break from studying. Perhaps consider inviting a group of friends over for some yoga.

There is no doubt that it will be harder for some and easier for others. But it's totally doable for everyone!

Just think of all the time you'll waste if you don't make time for your body: you will spend more time (and money) buying new clothes because you won't fit into your old ones. You will spend more time doing simple jobs such as mowing your lawn or carrying grocery bags from your car to your house because you aren't strong enough to do them quickly and easily. You'll spend more time being sick. That's right—*if you don't have physical activity in your life, you will spend eight days more per year being sick*. Think of how much time that will cost you.

To avoid all this (and get countless benefits), all you need to do is exercise three times a week for thirty minutes. That's ninety minutes per week, or six hours per month, or seventy-eight hours a year. In other words, you need to dedicate only the equivalent of about three days per year to exercise! Remember, though, that it has to be spread out over the year, not just three consecutive days of exercise.

Making a commitment to exercising regularly is the greatest health investment you will ever make in your entire life. If you were really sick, would you be too busy to see your doctor? If your son or daughter or a good friend were getting married, would you be "too busy" to go to the wedding? The fact of the matter is that you can't do *anything* without your body, and if your body is not up to the task, it doesn't matter how busy you think you are, you're not going to get what you want.

MORE EXCUSES TO BE AWARE OF—AND TO CHANGE!

1. *I don't have the energy.*

   Guess what? Exercising gives you more energy. You're going to be far less tired if you are active. Your lack of energy is likely because you are not active, not the other way around.

2. *I'll hurt myself.*

   If you have been inactive for a long time, begin exercise very slowly and build up gradually. It's not necessary to jump into things that are beyond your capability. Regular exercise strengthens your muscles and bones, so the more you exercise, the less likely you are to get hurt. People who don't exercise have more aches and pains than those who do. You could also do a few sessions with a personal trainer.

3. *I have to be so dedicated—it takes a lot of will power.*

   It doesn't. All you need is thirty minutes, three times a week. This can get you to 95 percent of your maximum fitness within six months. Just show up!

4. *I can't afford expensive exercise equipment.*
   You don't need any. Many exercises do not require
   special equipment. Some physical activities, such as
   walking or running, don't require any equipment other
   than a good pair of shoes and comfortable clothing.
   And if you happen to be a member of a fitness club, all
   the "expensive equipment" is there for you. You don't
   need to own any of it yourself.

5. *I can't afford to join a fitness club.*
   There is a fitness club for everyone. Most range in
   price from $20 to $60 per month and have a variety
   of membership options from which to choose. If you
   think about that, it's no different than eating out at a
   nice restaurant once a month or buying a cup of coffee
   every day.

6. *I don't look good in shorts.*
   Then don't wear them! You can exercise wearing
   sweatpants and other loose-fitting clothes.

7. *I'll start tomorrow.*
   Ah yes, but tomorrow never comes, does it? There is
   only today.

NEVER UNDERESTIMATE THE POWER OF OPTIMISM

My grandmother Gwendolyn Clarke used to love to tell the story of her first model-T car, which she dubbed The Optimist. The car cost $75, and after only three half-hour lessons, she took it on the road. "Possibly the 'optimist' applies to the driver as well as the car!" she wrote in one of her newspaper columns.

That made me think: each and every one of us is the "driver" of our own body. Our brain is the driver, and the energy generated by physical activity is the fuel. When you feel good and have lots of energy, you are naturally more optimistic. If you're sluggish and lethargic because you've been a couch potato for too long, you see life in a more pessimistic frame of mind. With high energy, obstacles become challenges that we can meet. With low energy, we call them problems. With high energy, we say, "Yes I can!" With low energy we say, "I don't think so." Realize that when it comes to your body, you are both driver and car. So choose to become the "optimist driver."

DO THIS

Implement some body- and mind-affirming practices over the next thirty days. Here are some suggestions:

- strength training
- massage
- sex
- contemplation/meditation
- breathing exercises
- walking
- running
- stretching in the shower
- dancing
- a group exercise class

Make sure your list of possibilities is longer than your list of excuses.

IT'S NEVER TOO LATE

A man came up to me one day and said, "I'm sixty years old. I can't do what I did when I was younger. It's been ages since I've exercised, so I'm thinking it's too late for me."

I asked him, "Well, you're not dead yet, are you? You're walking around and talking. Why do you think it's too late to start exercising?" I told him that the fact he was thinking about exercise indicated that the will was there. He just needed to believe it would be worth a try.

Did you know?

A 2006 study reported in *The Journal of the American College of Cardiology* found that when sedentary adults in their sixties and seventies walked at the same pace as people in their thirties, they had to use more oxygen. But after going through a six-month exercise program—they walked, biked, and stretched three days a week—the older adults improved the efficiency of their heart and lungs. In fact, the seniors' exercise efficiency increased by 30 percent, compared to only 2 percent among the younger exercisers. Wow!

It's *never* too late to start exercising. If you're fifty, sixty, or even eighty-five and you haven't exercised in a long time (or never have), you can still start. And you will see the benefits. Amazingly, I get the same question from people even in their teens or twenties. They, too, think it's too late. It's not! Should you try? You should. Will it work for you? It will.

DO THIS

Follow Patch's "One More" rule. For one month, increase your physical activity by one more unit per week, whether in minutes or numbers. For example, if you can walk for five minutes one week, the next week walk for six minutes. Then make it seven, and so forth. If you can swim ten laps, add one more per week. If you're working with weights, increase the number of repetitions or pounds by one every week throughout the month. You can carry this on for a very long time—imagine the effect this will have on you after a year of adding "just one more" onto some of your key physical activities.

CHAPTER 18

GO FOR THE LAUGHS

Picture a time when you doubled over with laughter and tears ran down your cheeks. We all know how absolutely wonderful that feels, during and after—laughter is one of nature's greatest gifts. A sense of humor is worth its weight in gold, or should I say it's worth *your* weight in gold (your healthy weight, of course!). Remember the endorphins we talked about earlier? Laughter is another major way to release endorphins in your body. There simply is no downside to laughter.

First of all, laughter is very magnetic. We want to spend time with people who make us laugh (and who think our jokes are funny!). When you allow laughter into your life, you are contributing to your health and the health of others.

Laughing is one of the best stress-busters. When we're in a "fight or flight" state, we release stress hormones into our body that increase our heart rate and blood pressure. Laughter neutralizes "fight or flight" residual stress by actually helping to reduce the stress hormones.

Have you ever been really nervous about something? Perhaps you're giving a presentation at work and you've got stage fright. Then a colleague comes along and says something that makes you laugh. After you've had that good laugh, you notice that you're not feeling quite so nervous. Or maybe you've included a funny story in your presentation and when you tell that story, your audience laughs. Their laughter makes your fear abate. You realize that your presentation really is going to be all right.

Did you know?

Laughter can alleviate pain. The pioneering work of mind/body scientist Norman Cousins showed the soothing effect of laughter. In his landmark book, *Anatomy of an Illness*, Cousins describes how he used laughter as part of his treatment for a rare spinal disease. Just ten minutes of laughter gave him two hours pain-free.

And guess what? Laughter is exercise! When we laugh, our diaphragm, abdomen, and facial, and back muscles all contract. There is wisdom in the phrase *laughing your ass off*. Not only is laughter an "inner massage" for all your organs, it burns calories too. When you laugh, you're getting a mini-workout.

Laughter can be an important part of a wellness program. In fact, upon discovering the healing effects of laughter, some teachers in India started laughter circles in their classrooms. The first thing children in their classrooms do in the morning is stand up and laugh for two minutes. I'd like to see that in all schools and workplaces. There is also a form of yoga called Laughter Yoga that has become quite popular all over the world.

DO THIS

If you get home from your workout and still feel the need to watch some TV, choose a comedy or a funny movie. Every day, find something to laugh about. Anyone can do this: My buddy Andy MacLaren sends me funny emails every couple of days, even though he has a serious financial job, and I think that's part of why he's so successful. Try it! Or if you get together with friends to go for a walk, before you start out, laugh for one full minute together. Sure, your crabby neighbor next door might think you're all crazy, but you know what? Laughter is contagious, so before you know it, your curmudgeonly neighbor will be laughing too.

30 MINUTES TO THE REAL SEXY, SMART, AND STRONG

We've been talking about how exercise improves your self-image and makes you feel energetic and full of life. We've talked about how exercise enhances your brain power and improves your mood. Now we need to focus on exercise's ability to give you physical strength, health, and endurance! I want you to pass this on to your family and friends. Why? Because one of the keys to being sexy, smart, and strong is the *strong* part of the equation.

You now know that you can get in shape by being physically active for thirty minutes, three times a week. Part III will show you how to take action. Exercise routines generally focus on either a cardiovascular workout or a strength workout. During the course of your week, you need to vary your program between these two, and stretching, warming up, and cooling down are important in order to protect against muscle strain and avoid muscle stiffness or soreness. Here are a few basics:

- Cardio exercise is movement that works your heart and lungs.
- Strength training is exercise that works targeted muscles in your body.
- Stretching is the act of positioning your body in order to lengthen a specific muscle.

Part III will tell you why you need to do all three of the above and how to integrate them into your life. While some of you may prefer lifting weights and others running on a treadmill, you still need a balanced approach that includes all three aspects of fitness. Here are some initial suggestions:

1. It helps to choose physical activities that you really enjoy. Do you like to dance? Many group exercise classes involve dance steps. You can learn all the latest hot salsa steps or move to the rhythms of jazz or rock. Do you enjoy mindful focus? You can explore BodyFlow, yoga, or tai chi, which include meditative elements within the physical movements. BodyPump™ classes are among the most popular (they are in more than twelve thousand clubs worldwide) for strength and cardio combined. Do you love being in water? Try an aqua fitness class. Love being outdoors? So walk— enjoy the clouds, snow, sunshine, rain. Choose window shopping or nature—just move it!

2. Even with exercise activities that have a repetitive quality such as running or walking, there are ways you can make it more entertaining. You can watch TV, listen to CDs, or read. You can ask friends to join you. If your friend is on the treadmill or cross-training beside you in the fitness club, you can talk, tell jokes, discuss the daily news or the neighborhood gossip. Also, try just moving and simply focusing on the movement itself. This is very relaxing.

3. Music is a huge motivator. Take an IPod or MP3 player along with you when you exercise. Plus, if you're going for a daily walk or run outside, do it in different locations for variety, and turn the music off in order to enjoy listening to nature. Change your route, or do it in reverse. Look forward to hearing the birds and feeling the sun or rain on your face.

4. Whether you are doing cardio or strength exercises, don't make it harder than it needs to be. One reason people hesitate to exercise is that they think they need to do really *hard* exercise in order for it to work, which is a turnoff for many. Maybe they don't enjoy heavy sweating, or feeling out of breath. The great news is that we now know that you don't need *vigorous* exercise to be fit and healthy, you simply need *moderate* exercise. Unless you're an athlete in training, moderate is more than enough. Good enough!

Don't tell me that you don't enjoy physical activity. That's just an excuse, a way of procrastinating; it's your good old subconscious mind messing with your intentions to be in good health. You can do it! You really can. Say *yes* to your body!

CHAPTER 19

LET'S CHAT ABOUT CARDIO

You've looked forward to your group exercise class all day. You find your spot on the floor, smile at the person next to you, and turn your eyes to the instructor. The music starts—it's a blend of Latin music and dance moves known as Zumba, a craze sweeping the fitness world. Watching the instructor's feet, you follow the beat! Throughout the hour-long class you dance the cha-cha, merengue, mambo, hip-hop—even belly dance. It's impossible to hear this music and not start moving. As the class progresses and your awareness of your body is heightened, you feel your heart beating and you feel some burn in your calves and hips (which might not have swayed that much in years). It just feels so good! As we progress through Part III, remember, cardio exercise can be a lot of fun.

Did you know?

Dancing can be a fantastic cardiovascular exercise—think of the last wedding where you danced for ten songs straight (or the equivalent of thirty to forty minutes of non-stop movement). Dancing is a wonderful form of exercise because it involves all of your body's major muscle groups, thereby giving your entire body a workout.

I've heard a lot of people say, "I don't dance." But you do. Your own "dance" or rhythm if you prefer, is attached to the way you drive, golf, run, swim, or walk. You don't have to be a hip-hop performer to get it. Whether you realize it or not, you've already got awareness of your rhythm. Being aware of your internal rhythm, your real dance, makes life that much better! Best of all—it's fun *and* sexy!

Keeping your heart and lungs strong is crucial to your overall health—and that is why getting cardiovascular exercise is so important.

In simple terms, the heart and lungs work together, and the blood, heart, and blood vessels form the cardiovascular system. They work together to deliver oxygen and nutrients to your body. Your lungs take the oxygen from the air and deposit it into the bloodstream. The heart is your pump, causing your blood to flow through the body by way of arteries and veins.

Cardiovascular exercise makes your heart and lungs work more efficiently, which means that your heart doesn't have to work as hard. This translates into you feeling less tired and having more energy. You'll also get a lower resting heart rate.

Why would you want your resting heart rate to go down? Because a lower resting heart rate signifies a more fit heart. The lower it is, the easier the load on your heart. The average North American resting heart rate is seventy-six beats per minute (with some difference between men and women). With regular activities that work your cardiovascular system, you can get your resting heart rate down. (Some athletes achieve heart rates in the thirties!)

Did you know?

A good way to figure out your resting heart rate is to check your pulse for one minute in the morning before you get out of bed. You can do this by locating the radial artery in your wrist or the large carotid artery in your neck. Be sure to use your index finger and your middle finger together to do this. Count how many beats in ten seconds and multiply that number by six. That gets your resting heart rate. Try this for five days in a row to get used to it and give you a reliable baseline. Heart rate watches and straps can help too.

The really neat thing about cardiovascular exercise is that there are so many activities to choose from. Here are some suggestions:

1. Go for regular walks. Start walking at a comfortable pace, then gradually work your way up (walk faster and for longer). If you swing your arms while you're walking, this will give your heart a better workout.
2. Jog at a moderate pace.
3. Ride a bicycle indoors or outdoors.
4. Go ice skating or cross-country skiing.
5. Inline skate.
6. Dance anywhere, anytime.
7. At a fitness club you can try treadmills, step machines, stationary cycles, or elliptical trainers (also referred to as cross-trainers) for a low-impact cardiovascular workout.

8. Try a group exercise class. You'll be boosted by the energy of the others in the class and it's a lot of fun.
9. Swim.
10. Play a recreational team sport such as hockey, basketball, soccer, or tennis.

DO THIS

This week (and if possible, every week thereafter), do one of these four things:

1. Walk or jog.
2. Go to a group fitness class that has dance moves— Latin, jazz, or hip-hop, you've got the moves!
3. Swim some laps in a local pool.
4. Walk five flights of stairs at least once a week.

CHAPTER 20

HOW DOES STRENGTH TRAINING WORK?

You need strength in order to enjoy a good life. By that I mean that strong muscles remove the obstacles, pain, and distress that can come from being weak. Strength training stabilizes the joints in your body by building up the muscles that support your bones—in other words, it helps protect your skeleton from injuries. It increases bone density and helps fine motor coordination (such as holding a pen) and gross motor coordination (such as kicking a soccer ball). You need strength for everyday things—carrying a suitcase or a bag of groceries, or lifting your child. It is also one of the very best ways to lose weight and improve your posture.

Did you know?

Strength training will not make you look bulky (unless you actually set out to become a body builder). Sometimes women express some concern about strength training. They may see it as something men are more drawn to, or they fear that they will end up looking "too muscular." "I don't want to look like a female body builder," they'll say. Fair enough. It takes tremendous, sustained effort to develop muscles "like a body builder," not to mention the dedication needed to achieve that level of leanness. By contrast, when you use strength training for firming your arms (for example), it will actually make you appear leaner, stronger ... dare I say, sexier!

The encouraging news is that no matter how old you are, the body responds positively to strength training. A short time ago I read an article in a national newspaper with the headline "GRANDPA GETS RIPPED." It was about a sixty-year-old dentist who became a competitive all-natural bodybuilder. In 2007, the World Natural Sports Organization had forty-four competitors older than sixty years!

Did you know?

From the age of twenty, you will lose about five to seven pounds (two to three kilograms) of muscle every decade you don't exercise (assuming you had some strength to begin with). That means that your metabolism—the breakdown of food and its transformation into energy—becomes less efficient as you age.

Your metabolism slows, meaning your body does not burn as much fat as it once did simply because you have less muscle. The good news is that current research at Boston University backs up the notion that stronger muscles equal a better metabolism. If you strength train, you'll add lean muscle mass back on. This is good. You can turn it around!

The key to strength training is that *all* your major muscle groups benefit from slow strength exercises. Why slow? Because you work the muscle better. Also, when you try to heave or throw a weight around quickly, you increase the potential for injury. If you exercise slowly and fully contract your muscle through the whole range of motion, you dramatically reduce any chance of injury. By not heaving the weight against gravity or cheating through those tougher spots, you use the muscle group you want to strengthen fully.

One of the easiest ways to do strength training is in a fitness club that has a wide variety of strength training equipment. Options include:

1. **Circuit training.** It's simple, easy to learn, and pretty well impossible to get hurt. Circuit training involves using six to twelve different pieces of strength training equipment. On each piece of equipment you will perform one set (eight to twelve repetitions) of the exercise. A good measure of whether you are choosing the right weight for you is that your muscles should tire after twelve repetitions. Each piece of equipment works a different group of muscles, and you can control the amount of weight—starting gradually and building as you progress. These machines have diagrams as well to show you how to correctly position your body for the best results. Have a club professional demonstrate how to coordinate your breathing. Simply put: exhale as you lift a weight; inhale as you lower the weight, preparing yourself for the next exertion.

   It's a good idea to exercise the large muscle groups first, working toward the small muscle groups. Start with a leg extension machine. This will strengthen the front of your thighs, known as your quadriceps. For the back of your thighs, known as your hamstrings, you can use another machine to perform what is known as a hamstring curl. Then continue by following the strength machine circuit to strengthen all the rest of your body. If you haven't done strength training before, starting with these machines helps to ensure you have good form and are doing the exercises safely and effectively.

2. **Free weights.** You can choose free weights (as opposed to a piece of strength training equipment) for use at home or in a fitness club. Plates in standard weights such as 2.5, 5, 10 pounds (1, 2, and 4.5 kilograms) and up are loaded on each end of the barbell, depending on what level you choose for your workout. Do a squat with a barbell for your leg strength. When you do a chest press, if you do it slowly you involve your chest muscles, your biceps, triceps, and shoulder muscles. You can work your whole chest in one exercise! Free weights function the same as weights attached to a pulley but give you the advantage of being able to work out anywhere and at any angle.

Did you know?

Your *total* time of continuous exercise should be about twenty minutes, and continuous strength training exercise is also cardiovascular exercise. That means that strength training is also exercise that helps improve the efficiency of your heart and lungs.

STRENGTH TRAINING AT HOME

I often get asked, "Is it possible to strength train at home? What if I can't get to a club or if I prefer to do it privately, without equipment?" The answer is yes, you can definitely strength train at home. Keep in mind, though, that training at home may not yield results as fast or as efficiently as when you would do it at a fitness club, but if you're dedicated and disciplined to do it at home, it does work!

Here are two excellent strength training exercises you can do anywhere—in your living room, your family room, your bedroom. Get started with these today:

1. Stand with your back to a chair. Cross your arms over your chest and squat down to where the seat of the

chair is (without touching it). Then stand up. Do this ten times (one set of ten). Two days later, do a set of ten again. Remember, the stronger you are, the more slowly you will be able to do this exercise, so take your time. "Safe, slow and strong" is the motto I use for strength training. That's not too hard, is it? It's very do-able—and you've just worked most of your lower body!

2. A second simple strength training exercise is the on-your-knees pushup. Instead of having your whole body extended, as for the traditional pushup, you start on your knees. Make sure your wrists are directly under your shoulders, and contract your stomach muscles to keep your abdomen strong and stable. Start with a set of ten and do this every other day. As you grow stronger, do the pushups more slowly. When you begin to feel you've gained more endurance, stop using your knees and go into a full pushup stance for the set of ten. You've just worked the upper half of your body and your core!

Just doing these two exercises will go a long way to making you stronger. Something this simple will get you started and help you experience the benefits of increased strength. Try it—you'll begin to feel a lot better!

DO THIS

Go slow, do less, get more. Instead of doing twenty pushups, try two to five executed slowly. Spend one minute doing pushups slowly, regardless of the number. Then wait for two days and try again.

AND DO THIS: Consider hiring a personal trainer to help you establish a strength training program. A personal trainer can not only advise you about every aspect of your strength routine, he or she is also there to encourage you, cheer you on, and motivate you. One really neat way to benefit from strength training and increase your social activity is to do strength training in a small group. Get your friends together and share the cost of a personal trainer. This is both cost-effective and a really fun way to get strong!

CHAPTER 21

HOW CARDIO AND STRENGTH TRAINING WORK TOGETHER

Now that you understand the basics of cardiovascular exercise and strength training, I want to talk about how these two types of exercise complement each other.

Your weekly exercise routine depends primarily on your goals. Let's say that you are a forty-seven-year-old woman and you want to strengthen your back because your job requires that you spend most of your day sitting at a desk and, as a result, your back is not getting enough movement. A couple of strength training sessions per week targeting your core muscles (trunk or middle section of your body) and one cardio session for a well-rounded dose of physical activity would help you tremendously. How much do you need to do? Twenty to thirty minutes at a time—easy to fit in.

Let's take a different goal. Say you are a young man. Due to several years of inactivity, you have gained twenty-five pounds. Your primary goal is weight loss. Here, strength training is a very effective way to shed pounds. Just the act of building up your lean muscle assists with burning off calories. It's a misconception that strength training will give you great big hulking muscles. It can, if you are a mesomorph body type and devote most of the day to lifting weights. But for most of us, the result is a lot more subtle in appearance but big in benefits. You can counteract osteoporosis (loss of bone density), which can affect both sexes; replace muscle mass lost as you age; and fundamentally help your body be strong enough for daily living. You'll look really good—strong and lean.

Did you know?

You learned earlier on how to find your resting heart rate. If you choose, you can check with your physician or personal trainer for more information on your *training* heart rate (the level of intensity at which you should exercise to really work your heart and lungs) and how to periodically check your pulse to see if you have reached your training heart rate. Go to www. goodlifefitness.com for a detailed description of how to get your training heart rate.

In both of these cases, your goal will dictate whether your focus is a strength workout or a cardiovascular workout. Either way, though, you still need both to some degree. In all cases, it's the regularity that's important. Some people ask, "Okay, Patch, if three times a week is good, what about five times a week?" Well, yes, you could get better results going five times a week for three or four months. Working out three times a week, you'd get the same results within six months as you would get doing it five times a week for four months. For most people it doesn't matter if it takes five months or six months. What I'm after here is to have you *do this for the rest of your life*. I want you to see that fitting exercise into your weekly schedule is doable. If you haven't been inclined to do regular activity all your life, don't go to the extreme. You'll feel overwhelmed and then you'll stop, and I don't want you to stop! Just do it regularly three times a week for twenty to thirty minutes.

DO THIS

Figure out whether you are more interested in cardio exercise or strength training. Then add in the other so that you've got a good combination. Schedule when you'll do your three times a week regimen for the first two months. Halfway through the second month, schedule in months three and four. Halfway through the fourth month, put the times for months five and six on your calendar. By now the "three times a week" will have become a habit, and that's a great habit to have!

CHAPTER 22

WORKOUT ESSENTIALS: WARMING UP, STRETCHING, AND COOLING DOWN

You've decided to include exercise in your life. That's great! However, in your eagerness to reap the full benefits of your exercise time, don't neglect three very important components: the warm-up, stretching, and the cool-down.

THE WARM-UP

In the warm-up phase, you're revving yourself up, anticipating the exhilarating feeling you'll get when you're in the intensity phase of your exercise routine.

Warming up involves stretching your muscles—crucial to helping your body adapt to the demands of exercise. It increases blood flow to the muscles. Jumping into a workout without preparing your body and your muscles can lead to muscle strain and soreness, and possibly even injury.

Did you know?

If you are older, are recovering from an injury, or have a condition such as arthritis, I recommend that you warm up for ten minutes instead of five.

Active stretching is geared for the warm-up phase. The idea is that you will be warming up all the major muscles, joints, and ligaments in your body in preparation for the exercise you are about to do. Listen to your body. For each of the warm-ups described below, you will be following your body's natural range of motion. For the first few repetitions of the movement, your natural range of motion will be smaller. As your body parts warm up, the range will be bigger. It is also important to understand that active stretching is continuous, fluid motion with no stopping until you are moving on to the next stretch. The following warm-up movements will raise your heart rate so you are preparing for both cardiovascular and strength workouts.

1. Thirty big but comfortable circles with each arm (like you're swimming the front crawl).

2. Thirty kicks with each leg. Swing your right leg from front to back, keeping your leg straight with your

knee slightly bent. Don't touch the floor. Then repeat with your left leg. (You might want to rest your hand on a balance bar or a table to do this.)

3. Thirty hip circles. Place your hands on your hips and rotate your torso as if you are swinging a hula hoop.

4. Warm up your knee area with a single-leg squat. Stand with your shoulder near a wall (in case you need some support or to balance with one hand). With your weight on one leg (just let the other hang loose), lower your body into a squat, just short of sitting down on a chair. Then stand straight again. Do this ten to fifteen times (one repetition) three times.

5. Cardio warm-up. Start easy on any cardio exercise machine. Gradually increase speed of movement and/or intensity. Do it for five minutes. At the end of your warm-up, you should feel "warm." Big surprise, hey?

These movements will take the blood away from your stomach and bring it more to the surface of your skin.

A STRETCHING LESSON FROM CATS

Many people seem to have forgotten that we're actually designed to be flexible. Flexibility improves with prolonged and careful stretching of the muscles, joints, fascia, and other connective tissues. That's why ballet dancers with training can place their leg on a ballet barre with ease.

We can learn by observing one of the most flexible animals—cats. If you watch cats, you'll see that they stretch all the time.

Have you ever seen a cat extend its paw up in the air and then turn it around? Try that—extend your arm and turn your palm up to the sky. You'll feel your forearm, shoulder, biceps, and triceps stretching, just from this simple action.

You've seen how cats arch their backs and put their head up in the air. That's actually fantastic for your back. In fact, it's a very well-known yoga pose called, not surprisingly, the Cat. Kneeling on hands and knees, curl your head toward your chest and round your back upward, then reverse by raising your head and sticking your butt up toward the sky. The Cat stretch helps your vertebrae and back muscles relax.

Here is a simple stretch for your shoulders and chest. Stand in a doorway and put your hands on each side of the doorway at shoulder height. Gently lean forward with your chest so that your arms are behind your chest and you are stretching your chest open. In our everyday activities we often spend a lot of time sitting at a computer or driving, and we're always bent forward, closing in our chest. The doorway exercise counterbalances this by opening up the chest.

Here is another easy stretch you can do: From a seated position, twirl your foot around in a slow, deliberate circle. This will stretch your foot and ankle muscles, and you'll also feel it in your calf muscles and even in your thighs. Now rotate in the opposite direction.

Doing some simple stretching activities at brief intervals during the day will help you maintain flexibility and gain relaxation. Try it in your car at a red light, during TV commercials, in meetings, or on the phone. Multitask in a good way!

Consider adding a purposeful ten to twenty minutes of stretching two or three times a week and use it as preparation for actual exercise. Cool-down stretching relaxes you so that you can get on with your day after your exercise period. A good way to experience the power of stretching is in a group exercise class such as BodyFlow, yoga, or tai chi.

Take a lesson from cats and stretch. It's said they have nine lives—maybe stretching adds one!

THE COOL-DOWN

Taking the time to cool down transitions your heart, lungs, and blood flow back toward a normal rate (i.e., non-exercising state). For example, you warmed up by stretching all the major parts of your body and by starting your walk slowly; then you did your brisk walk/jog for twenty to thirty minutes. Now you will finish off by cooling down. Particularly if you had an intense workout where you have kept your heart rate up, you will want to walk slowly for at least a few minutes—on a treadmill or outside, wherever you are. If you are de-conditioned (perhaps you haven't exercised in a while) or have higher than normal blood pressure, then this return to a slow walk for a few minutes is especially important before you sit down or lower your head. You can finish off with a few static stretches, if you want. Fitness clubs usually have a stretching area complete with diagrams. By investing a few minutes here, you will not have any soreness the next day! Or go to the GoodLife website, goodlifefitness.com, for more information on stretching.

Most injuries or muscle stiffness or soreness are the result of neglecting to warm up and cool down. I like to think of warm-ups and cool-downs as my own internal "coaches." You're switching your brain to active mode while also allowing it to relax and recover. It's an opportunity to check in with your body, see how it's feeling, and decide how hard you can push yourself today.

In the cool-down phase, you get to savor the feelings of well-being that permeate the body after exercise, to experience the effects of those wonderful endorphins, and to congratulate yourself on exercise well done. You can have confidence that you'll be invigorated, mentally rested, and will get more done faster. It's rejuvenating!

One of the best places to get used to good stretching and warming-up and cooling down techniques is a group exercise class. It's pretty hard to get the same instruction from a diagram or chart. Many fitness clubs offer free introductory passes on their websites, which is a great place to start.

DO THIS

Do three of the stretches I described in this chapter as part of your workouts over the next couple of weeks. They're easy! What are you waiting for?

CHAPTER 23

"NO PAIN, NO GAIN" IS FALSE

Let's talk about this "no pain, no gain" idea: it's garbage and totally untrue! The idea that exercise is somehow supposed to hurt is the number-one reason why people don't exercise (on top of feeling self-conscious while they exercise, which we talked about in Part II). Sometimes people say to me, "Well, I exercised today and I don't hurt anywhere. Is it working?" Of course it's working!

If you hurt the next day or later, you've pushed yourself too far, too quickly. In many cases, the best way to recover is to do the same exercises more slowly, and with less intensity and less weight. Add a proper warm-up and cool down. A hot shower or bath and a massage are also really great ways to relax and to take care of your body after a workout.

If you are experiencing discomfort or if a movement hurts while you are exercising, that is a signal to back off. Use the same common sense you do when you are eating. You eat enough to feel satisfied, not totally full, right? If you stuff yourself, your gut hurts and you feel like a slug later and even into the next day. Overexercise and you'll feel the same. Life is actually a marathon, not a sprint. The fit turtle wins the race.

Largely the "no pain, no gain" myth comes from high-level athletics or the military. We see how elite athletes push themselves to the limits of their endurance, and somehow that has become synonymous with "exercise." But most of us are not training for the Olympics! Modeling a fitness routine after the programs followed by elite athletes (or, more to the point, mimicking how we *think* they work out) just isn't useful.

Did you know?

When you first begin exercising after a long sedentary period in your life, your muscles are going to feel the effects. So you may feel the stretch, but it should be a good kind of feeling. This is a natural reaction to your muscles being (safely) worked out, and it's entirely normal.

If you're exercising and feeling real pain, you're doing it too hard. The idea is not to make your muscles hurt; it's to make your muscles grow stronger and to make you feel more alive. However, if it hurts so much that you are really uncomfortable, then you're working too hard. Back off on the weight, the intensity, or both. Build up slowly.

Likewise, if you feel exhausted an hour after exercise, you're doing too much. Exercise is supposed to give you energy and strength, not take it away. Again, if you're just starting exercise for the first time, you may feel a bit tired, but it's a satisfying kind of tired. It's the kind of tired you feel when you've been out dancing and having a good time. There's a big difference between that sensation and real fatigue. Build to a "good enough" slowly and steadily.

The "no pain, no gain" myth has got to be turfed out of your mind. Don't buy into it. Replace that idea with a picture in your mind of a stronger you, with great energy, better posture, and an improved shape—sexy, smart, and strong!

DO THIS

After you exercise, take a couple of minutes to evaluate your body. Do you hurt anywhere? A couple of hours later, take stock again ... do you feel any pain now? (Sometimes the pain from overexertion shows up a few hours later.) If you notice that you're really sore, back off a bit the next time around. But don't stop!

CHAPTER 24

GET OTHERS INVOLVED

Very often when people get into regular physical activity and begin to see and feel the benefits, they want to tell others about it. They'll say, "Okay, Patch, I'm totally into this exercise thing. I've lost some weight, I've got a lot more energy, and I feel really good! Now how do I convince my spouse, my kids, or my friends to do it?"

The answer is to find a way to share your enthusiasm without becoming preachy about it. The best way to influence people is to set a good example yourself, so that they learn from your *actions* more than from your words. When your family and friends see you exercising and become aware of the "new energetic you," they will naturally gravitate toward what you are doing. They'll think, "Maybe I should do what you're doing, to get what you've got."

On top of modeling good health, you can also find encouraging ways to include others in your exercise. If you go for regular walks, bring a friend or family member with you. If you're going to the fitness club, invite them to come along and check the place out.

Another thing you can do is talk about what exercise has done for you. Keep it personal, rather than telling others what it should be for them. Say things such as "My back doesn't hurt anymore" or "I've lost a couple of belt sizes (or dress sizes)" or "I really enjoyed going dancing the other night—two years ago I wouldn't have lasted ten minutes." I have also heard people say, "My skin is so much clearer and softer now. Many of my facial lines have smoothed out." People will soon become curious about what your secret is.

Being a "gentle advocate" of everyday exercise is great as well. At work, you could be the one who says, "It's only three floors up! Let's walk up the stairs instead of taking the elevator." You might get some glares or raised eyebrows, but just maybe some of your co-workers will agree to join you on the stairs. If you have a meeting outside your office and it's not too far away, suggest that people walk to the meeting rather than drive. Stand up at intervals during some of your meetings. All these things encourage people who are important to you to try physical activity for themselves. And who benefits? You all do!

Another really neat way to be an advocate for fitness is to become involved in some of the many charitable events that integrate some form of fitness activity. There are events such as runs for cancer or arthritis or children's centers, or swim-a-thons, dance-a-thons, walks, bicycle rides—all for a myriad of great causes. Getting involved with an activity-oriented charitable event is a great way to meet new friends and enjoy socializing as well as getting fit.

These types of events are always looking for volunteers. You can get involved both by helping to organize the event and by doing the activity. You'll feel doubly good! You're doing something that benefits your own health and well-being, and you're contributing to a good cause, something that can make a difference to a lot of people.

Whether it's in your own family, at your workplace, or out in the community, you can be an ambassador for physical activity. It's not enough just to "get the message out" that exercise is good for us. What we need are people who will model what that is like—healthy vital people who are out there enjoying physical activity and who can show us all just how easy it is!

Did you know?

Charitable events involving some form of physical activity are growing in popularity across North America. Almost every community has at least one. If your community doesn't have one, then make it a family outing to drive to a nearby town or city to participate in an event happening there.

WORK OUT WITH A PARTNER

One of the best ways to stay motivated in physical activity is to work out with a partner or friend. Sometimes people say to me, "Patch, I'd love to work out with my husband (or wife or boyfriend/girlfriend), but he/she is in much better shape than I am. So how can I do this?"

1. If your exercise buddy is more fit than you are, or vice versa, find ways to complement each other. For example, if your partner likes to inline skate, and he or she inline skates really fast and you're the slower one, get on a bicycle. Your partner inline skates. You bike beside your partner. You both end up getting exercise—together.

2. Or let's say that your partner is an experienced weightlifter and you're not that strong yet. You can

still strength train together because you can choose individual weights to work with. It doesn't matter how strong either of you are, both of you will need help on that last rep. So there's no reason your partner can't help you get your last rep even though you might be doing half as much weight.

3. Consider taking fitness classes together. In group exercise, people go at their own pace. So it doesn't matter in that setting whether your partner is faster or stronger than you. You'll both have fun.

4. Let's say your friend runs faster or likes to go farther than you do. Then join them for the last twenty to thirty minutes of their run. Or run on a track together so you keep seeing each other. You can alternate your running with some walking and still end together!

5. If you ski or snow board, take the chairlift together.

6. Golf is easy to do together, as is lane swimming. Bicycle for two.

7. Sometimes it's fun to purposely pick an activity the other person is better at, in order to stretch yourself. A good stretch class for the weightlifter is a perfect example of trying something different. That's beneficial socially, physically, and intellectually!

Be creative. There are lots of different ways to do the same activity. In some cases, the person who started off as the novice partner in the activity will catch up with or surpass the more experienced one. Maybe this is a lesson for relationships in general—learning to adapt to each other and grow with each other. Let physical activity help you with that.

UNEXPECTED BENEFITS OF GROUP EXERCISE

One of my club members, Scott, got a wake-up call when his colleague died suddenly of cardiac arrest at the age of thirty-nine. Scott had been losing his motivation for exercise, but when his colleague died, he decided he had to get back to it. He wanted something different, so in 2004, he started participating in group exercise classes. All of a sudden he was excited to go to the club. That same year he went through more personal losses when both his uncle and his father died. Scott credits the "group ex" classes with helping him maintain his equilibrium. The social aspect of group exercise helped Scott feel a sense of connection with others. In 2005, Scott decided to train as a BodyFlow instructor. His training program gave him the confidence to get up in front of people. Not only was he getting the physical benefits of group exercise, he was also leading other people to experience those same benefits.

DO THIS

The best way to help someone you care about is by inviting them to an activity you both love to do together. Say you and your best friend are avid golfers. A little sport-specific exercise (in this case, something that would develop your back and arms) can improve your game and help you finish strong rather than sore!

CHAPTER 25

FAMILY FITNESS

It's long been my contention that the earlier you get into the exercise habit, the more likely it is to stick with you throughout your lifetime. If you are an adult exerciser—whether beginner or advanced—consider taking the time to be an exercise role model for children. Set an example, both by exercising yourself *and* by playing a sport with kids.

Children should be exercising every single day for no less than thirty to sixty minutes—no if's, and's, or but's about it. Why? For their health, for their long life, for their brain power. Study after study has shown that exercise improves oxygen flow to all parts of the body, and that includes the brain. These same studies show that exercise improves functions such as productivity and concentration. If we don't make it possible for children to access regular physical activity in a low-cost way, we are robbing them of their health potential and learning capacity. It's like running a six-cylinder car on one cylinder. Childhood obesity is a serious problem in both the United States and

Canada, with most studies agreeing that more than
40 percent of our children are overweight.

If you didn't exercise as a child, you put yourself at higher
risk of, among many other things, becoming overweight.
If your child is overweight, when he or she grows to
adulthood, there is the risk of many chronic diseases,
particularly high blood pressure and heart disease. I was
alarmed at a recent news story on Canadian television
reporting that non-exercising children as young as eight or
nine years old are beginning to show signs of high blood
pressure. Other researchers have sounded the warning
that for the first time in recorded history, our children are
facing a shorter lifespan than their parents are!

Just having children play active games will do wonders
for their health and their sense of well-being. For children,
fitness is play. In 1999, I founded the GoodLife Kids
Foundation to help kids and families learn the why and
how of staying fit, eating right, and feeling good. With
a little help, kids will do the rest. Running, jumping,
somersaulting—all these come naturally to kids. We
need our communities to be environments that keep kids
moving. Organizations such as Right to Play promote
children's health worldwide. It's the smart thing to do.
Our future depends on it.

WONDERFUL MOMENTS AND ADVENTURES

Getting fit with your kids can spark some of life's most memorable moments. Think of those precious weekends your family spends bicycling or building sandcastles. Or the dance recital your daughter spent weeks preparing for, leading up to the final night onstage. These are the moments we can all relate to—the physical activities that nourish our children's minds and bodies and add extra zest to our day-to-day lives.

There are also some big adventures, exciting opportunities to get fit as a family that may only come along once in a lifetime. Recently my eleven-year-old daughter, Tygre, and I had the opportunity to swim with the dolphins in Orlando, Florida. I will let Tygre tell you about it in her own words:

> The sky was very blue and it was a sunny day. The water was calm and a shade of turquoise different from our northern lakes in Canada. I love to swim, so I waded in with confidence up to my waist. I felt a great sense of excitement waiting in the slightly chilly water to meet the dolphins. There were about five of us, including my dad, and the same number of dolphins swimming around. Magically, before long one of the dolphins named Cindy sought us out and came over with a friendly nod of her

head. I stroked her, as instructed, behind her blow hole, touching her silky gray back. As with many animals, they love a gentle touch, but not on their faces. Cindy caused us to giggle in delight when she rolled over on her back and let us touch her white belly. She was a beautiful soft-gray color with a light-colored belly. It felt like she was happy to entertain us!

Dolphins are wonderful communicators and highly intelligent. Cindy performed for us with a variety of sounds. She mimicked the sound of a fishing reel winding in the catch. Too funny! Then it was time for my "ride." I grabbed hold of her dorsal fin (on her back) and one of her flippers at her side, and we were off. Cindy did a big loop into slightly deeper water, sliding through the clear waters. The sensation was wonderful! Faster than I could possibly swim and so smooth!

One thing I know for sure: I really want to return next year, if I am lucky, and repeat the whole experience. My dad does too!

Your family can have big adventures too—the only limit is your imagination. Don't mistake "big" experiences for something that costs a lot of money. For instance, perhaps someone in your family will be lucky enough to be one of the "ordinary citizens" chosen one day to carry the Olympic torch through your town! Remember though, you won't find chances to do something exciting sitting all day at your computer. Put yourself out there and go find your adventures!

FUELING UP AS A FAMILY

Grocery shopping for healthy foods is a wonderful family activity—and a great way to teach your children about nutrition. I believe there is a real art to grocery shopping. The grocery store is one of the greatest "inventions" of our society. You can go to one place to find meat, fruit, vegetables, dairy products, and foods from around the world to satisfy every taste. My own particular joy is the organic section. Many supermarkets have great organic departments where you can find food the way it was a hundred years ago, before pesticides and antibiotics entered the food chain. In my opinion, the more natural foods you can eat, the better!

Let's begin our trip to the supermarket. First of all, realize that grocery stores have invested in a lot of marketing. The companies that make groceries and the stores that sell them cater to people's desires (and even create those desires). Often it's the most attractive packaging or the most prominent display that inspires you to put food products in your shopping cart. So the first thing you have to do is learn to resist the intriguing displays and not impulse shop. I find it helps to shop after you have eaten to help contain yourself.

Always shop the perimeter first. Go right around the store's outside aisles before going down any other aisles. It's in the outside aisles where you find the fresh produce, the fresh meat, the fresh dairy products. I call the inside rows of supermarkets "sugar central." In the inside aisles you find all the packaged foods, which tend to have too much sugar or salt and food preservatives. I'm not saying that you shouldn't ever buy barbecue sauce or packaged foods, but most of your groceries should come from the outside aisles of the store.

If you follow my "once around the outside aisle" method, you'll end up with a lot more nutritious food in your shopping cart. It's also faster! This will help make your visits to the inner aisles more sporadic. As much as possible, buy fresh. That's one way you can taste the good life!

DO THIS

If you have children, gather them around the dining room table and plan to do something fun and active together. Let the kids choose the activity. If it's summer, it might be a picnic complete with family races. If it's winter, maybe they'll want to go tobogganing or skating. Plan an "adventure" out in the country. Make it a regular thing you do—let each of your children choose a favorite activity and then do it together as a family.

CHAPTER 26

EXERCISE IS YEAR-ROUND

All four seasons of the year offer great opportunities for exercise. Each season offers its own special variety—a nice bonus because it helps us stay engaged all year long.

FITNESS IN FALL

The fall is one of the best seasons to do outdoor activities. The cooler days are refreshing, there's still a lot of daylight, and it's an energetic time of year.

A hike in the woods and fields is great both for your camera and your body. Take your binoculars too, because wildlife can be very active at this time of year, especially early in the morning or just before sunset. For the inner naturalist in you, have some fun identifying the plants, birds, and animals. In the wild, I've seen moose, beaver, deer, black bears, coyotes, and wolves. The fish are still biting too—you just need to do a little research on the best fishing holes.

If you live in a fruit-growing area where there is an autumn harvest, you can go apple picking. Your arm muscles in particular can get a great strength workout from reaching up to pick the fruit. Carrying the full baskets to the checkout area and loading them into your car is exercise too!

If you have kids, raking leaves can be made into a game—building a really high pile of leaves and jumping into them. After the fun is over, have them help you bag them and take them to the curb.

Years ago, many communities held fall corn roasts. There were always outdoor games, races, and contests that got people moving around, having a great time together, and filling the air with laughter. If your community doesn't have a fall corn or wiener roast, then why not plan your own in your backyard or a nearby park? Everyone can pitch in with ideas and sporting equipment such as Frisbees, baseballs, or footballs.

Another thing about the fall is that it is a prime time for people to join fitness clubs. What a great idea to shed a few pounds so you have some wiggle room for the upcoming holiday feasting!

EXERCISING IN WINTER

There is something about winter that makes it one of my favorite times of the year. Skating, skiing, sledding, or snowshoeing are all things that you can only do in the winter. A couple of times a year I go heli-skiing with friends—a helicopter drops us into fresh powder at the top of the mountains in British Columbia. I love the feeling of sinking up to my armpits in the snow and then twisting and turning my way down a steep incline on my skis. I find myself laughing out loud as I ski, just from the sheer joy of it.

How do you dress for being active in the cold? Most important, keep your feet and hands dry, so invest in some good socks and gloves. You'll also need weather-sealed boots that keep your feet warm and allow them to breathe.

We lose a lot of body heat through our heads, so it's important to wear a hat. If the wind chill is strong, keep your head warm. The rest of your clothing should be multilayered because the weather can vary a lot in winter, as can your level of exertion. It's best to wear clothing made from "wick-away" material (absorbs sweat) next to your skin and then two or three more layers. That gives you the option to take some of it off if you need to.

And wear long underwear! People tend to get tight hamstrings and soreness from their legs getting cold. They are wearing lots on the upper body but not enough on the lower body.

If your physical activity involves wind and sun, don't forget sunscreen lotion and winter sunglasses.

Water is as essential in the winter as in the summer, yet often forgotten. Carrying water for any length of time need not present a problem. Simply use an insulated covering for your water bottle found at most outdoor stores.

SPRING TRAINING FOR SUMMER SPORTS

Popular sports such as golf, cycling, and running—great spring and summer sports—all benefit from sport-specific training. That means getting the required muscles in shape as well as paying attention to your cardio.

For example, if you are a golfer, you need total body conditioning to play your best game. Golf is a total-body activity. Let's take your swing for starters. For a good swing, your entire body has to be stable and strong. Strengthening your core will help your back and hips (essential in the swing). Legs get a workout from walking the course so ditch that golf cart, if possible. All golfers want their drive to go farther (straight is good too!) so think about how much better you would be at executing your swing if you were stronger, more balanced, and flexible.

Other physical activities to get started on in spring are cycling and running. Start by taking fifteen- to twenty-minute bike rides in your neighborhood. You will be able to tell very quickly if your bike needs adjustments or repairs. It's a great way to get reacquainted with the controls and the biomechanics of your body. It's a good idea to stretch your legs and back after each ride. Don't neglect the hamstrings! Now you're ready to increase the duration of your ride and maybe add a few hills. Hills are where it all happens! The farther you can get away from traffic and enjoy the outdoors, the better.

Many "learn to run" programs start in February and March. As spring goes on, there are more and more runs. Typically, you will walk for the majority of the time when you are just starting, and then running is introduced gradually. Of course you will start with appropriate stretching exercises. If you haven't run before, get some expert advice on footwear for your foot and body type. This will reduce the risk of injury.

Your spring prep time will pay off in the long run (pun intended!).

SUMMER: AHHH, THE BEACH

Do you know what I love about the summer? The beach!
Going barefoot, wrestling the waves, watching people in
the water—loads of fun.

When I go to the beach, I try to pay attention to the
essentials. Be sure to pack lotion with a good sunblock
and a hat and sunglasses so you will be comfortable and
able to spend more time outdoors. Shoes or sandals help
protect your feet when the sand gets too hot to walk
on. A beach umbrella is always a good idea to provide
some shade, and don't forget containers of water to stay
hydrated.

Did you know?

Heat exhaustion and heat stroke are caused by an
imbalance between water and your electrolytes—
sodium, potassium, and calcium. Heat exhaustion is
when your body's perspiration is unable to keep up
with heat stress. Heat stroke is a medical emergency
and must be treated immediately. Symptoms are
profuse sweating, pale or flushed skin, headache,
dizziness, elevated body temperature, rapid pulse, and a
feeling of weakness. If you have any of these symptoms,
get to a cooler place, take off excess clothing, sponge
the body with cooler water, and drink lots of water.

Get medical help right away. Drinking extra water in the summer is the best way to stay hydrated and reduce the risk of heat stroke.

Beaches lend themselves to more than just lying around on a towel. Beach volleyball is a fun game that's very social. It's also a great workout mainly because of the amount of jumping, which requires a lot of energy. If you are at the seashore, try surfing. If you have never surfed before, sign up for a couple of lessons. You might also want to try snorkeling, scuba diving, wind-surfing, kayaking—endless choices.

Freshwater lakes are popular for canoeing, water-skiing, and wakeboarding, as well as a good refreshing swim.

Enjoy your summer activities early in the morning or late in the afternoon to avoid the hottest time of the day. Wear loose-fitting clothing that is breathable, such as cotton. Choose light colors that won't absorb sunlight and—bonus—they won't attract as many bugs!

Take advantage of those long summer days to be sexy, smart, and strong!

DO THIS

Enjoy some season-specific exercise. Feel yourself in tune with the rhythm of nature as you allow your body to experience things that can only be experienced in the season you're in!

CHAPTER 27

WHEN YOU TRAVEL

I travel close to 200,000 kilometers (124,274 miles) a year—that's the equivalent of five times around the circumference of the world! So I have lots of travel stories to tell, but also lots of experience on beating jet lag and keeping your energy up. If I am presenting at a conference in Asia, for example, then I need to be on my game pretty much from the moment I arrive.

No matter where you travel, there is always going to be a way for you to include exercise in your schedule. Sometimes your travel activities *are* the exercise. For example, if you spend all day exploring a foreign city on foot, you're getting plenty of exercise. Or maybe you're going swimming or surfing as part of your travels. That's exercise too. If you're traveling on business where you'll be in meetings all day, or if your vacation includes visiting a lot of restaurants serving gourmet meals, you may need to focus more on the physical and not neglect it. So consider getting up early to exercise, no matter what time you go to bed.

UNEXPECTED BENEFITS TO
EXERCISING WHILE TRAVELING

The last time I was in Australia, I had a magical exercise experience. I had been out with friends until 1:30 a.m. My plane was leaving at 5:00 a.m. back to North America, but I still had to get my daily workout in—no way was I traveling a thirty-hour stretch without exercising first! So at 2:30 a.m. I went running. I don't normally run (it's hard with my arthritis) but that was the only physical activity available because we were in the country. So here I am running down the middle of a road in the middle of the night, no cars and very much alone. I heard a noise—*whomp!* Then thirty seconds later, *whomp* again. And I'm thinking, "Whoa, that's kinda loud and whatever it is sounds *big*!" I have a young St. Bernard that weighs more than one hundred and sixty pounds (seventy-three kilograms) and a horse that measures seventeen hands, so I know about big. Then I hear it again—*whomp!* I hear it ten or fifteen times, and all of a sudden I look to the side and there's a big red kangaroo right beside me, looking me straight in the eye. I'm six-foot-four (193 centimeters), but this animal looked huge! We stared at each other— each one of us as startled as the other. Then he hopped off with a *whomp* of his tail and a lot more spring in *his* step. (Or maybe it was a she, I couldn't tell.) That was pretty cool—a little reward from Mother Nature for being so dedicated to my workouts.

DO THIS

On your next vacation, come up with ways to take your workout with you. Many hotels and resorts have full-service fitness facilities. And most cities, and even many smaller towns, have fitness clubs or community facilities that would be happy to provide you with a guest pass. The Internet is a great tool for that kind of search. Just go to your favorite search engine and type in the location you are going to and the keywords *fitness clubs* or *health clubs*. You can also get advice from the hotel when you are making your reservation so you are ready to go when you arrive!

CHAPTER 28

EXERCISING WITH CHRONIC PAIN

Chronic conditions are very much a part of life, spanning all age groups. Regular exercise can reduce the risk of developing many limiting conditions such as heart disease and stroke, diabetes and arthritis. It also serves to reduce your risk of diseases, including many forms of cancer. For most conditions, exercise also helps you get better. For people with osteoporosis, for example, weight-bearing exercise has been shown to increase bone density. With few exceptions, most people can perform moderate exercise. It is always a good idea, however, to consult your doctor and discuss your exercise prescription before getting started on an exercise plan. In this way you can better understand and adjust your physical activity to accommodate any ongoing health issues you might have.

At age thirty-two, I had just won a major rowing competition when I woke up the next day to a body on fire. The bed sheets felt enormously heavy. I was soaked

in sweat and suffering unbearable pain. That day I went
from athlete to ancient. I felt instantly very old, fragile,
weak, unstable ... and all overnight. I was exhausted by
the pain, unable to sleep. I couldn't turn a doorknob. My
swollen hands and feet wouldn't work. I could barely
move. I was terrified. What was happening to me? Finally,
months later, after a lot of tests at the hospital, a doctor
said, "Patch, you've got rheumatoid arthritis."

After my diagnosis, the doctors told me not to exercise.
I obeyed them for a few weeks, but I was just getting
weaker. In my usual stubborn manner, I decided to go
ahead and exercise. I was supposed to be "Mr. GoodLife
Fitness"—I'd always told everyone else the answer was
exercise. It was time to follow my own prescription
because clearly bed rest was not working. When I got
back onto a stationary bicycle after just a few weeks
of inactivity and pain, I had to have someone help me
turn the wheels! After about six weeks, I could turn the
wheels myself. Then I had to have help with the weights,
and when I did the strength training everything hurt.
Gradually I began to notice an improvement.

With any chronic illness, you need to figure out how to be
as strong as you can be. I knew this from my background
in exercise physiology. You can adapt exercise so that
you can continue with regular physical activity. As the

population ages, chronic conditions such as arthritis will become more and more of a health issue. I urge you to find your quality of life in any way you can, no matter what your condition. Don't give in. Don't give up. Just keep doing it.

Did you know?

The Arthritis Society now advocates exercise, citing benefits such as lessening of pain and improvement in flexibility and mood. They also state that activity aids in keeping joints healthy, since movement helps cartilage absorb nutrients.

DO THIS

If you have been diagnosed with a chronic condition, make a point of talking to your doctor about how exercise can help you. Ask your doctor to refer you to a physiotherapist or personal trainer who can help you design and maintain an exercise program that's right for you. It might also be a good idea to ask the doctor giving you the advice whether he or she incorporates fitness into his or her own life!

CHAPTER 29

OH, MY ACHING BACK

Back pain is the most common physical complaint people bring to doctors and chiropractors. The National Institute of Arthritis and Musculoskeletal and Skin Diseases reports that eight out of ten people will experience back pain at some point in their life. It's a major reason why people stay off work or quit exercising. If you're suffering with back pain, your sense of strength and vitality is reduced. You feel fragile. Life is compromised. You feel powerless. Out of control. And you hurt … a lot.

What causes back pain? Very simply, for the most part, it's muscle weakness brought on by sedentary living— 80 percent to 90 percent of back pain is caused by weak muscles in your back and abdomen. This weakness sneaks up on you as you age. If you haven't been staying in shape through regular exercise, eventually things that used to be simple become harder. One day you twist in a certain way and *ouch*! In common parlance, you "put your back out." In some cases, as with a herniated disc, for example, if your back pain is causing nerve pain or numbness down your legs, it's important to see a doctor.

There are some key things to help your back. First, you need to strengthen your body's core, which includes your abdominals and your back muscles. There is equipment in fitness clubs as well as personnel who can help you develop a series of exercises aimed at increasing your core strength. It is essential to a healthy back. There are also some things you can do just at home.

Another way to help your back is to strengthen the rest of your body. Why? So you don't put extra strain on your back! You see, the back is the fulcrum, axis, or center of gravity for your body. If your legs, arms, chest, back, or shoulders are too weak when you are performing a movement such as lifting, the energy gets transferred to your back to compensate for that weakness. Too much compensating strains the back. So ideally spend twenty minutes, two to three times a week, keeping your whole body strong.

DO THIS

Lie on the floor on your back with your arms at your sides and knees bent. Pull your abdominals in, squeeze your buttocks, and lift your hips off the ground, hold for one to two deep breaths, lower, and repeat five to eight times. Also include some basic abdominal curl-ups in your exercise program. One great place to learn how to effectively and safely perform this exercise is by attending a group fitness class.

CHAPTER 30

WHAT'S THE BEST EXERCISE EXPERIENCE YOU'VE EVER HAD?

That's a question I like to ask people who have pushed their physical boundaries when it comes to exercise. What's the physical activity that really taught them something important? Was there a life-changing experience that they never thought possible, that they did and will never forget? For a mother and her fifteen-year-old daughter that I know, it was riding horseback for six days, 110 miles (177 kilometers), on their own, across rugged terrain in Ireland. Seeing the pristine beaches, the countryside in forty shades of green, the seals gliding in the tidal waters—not to mention the mother-daughter bonding that happened!—more than made up for the physical discomfort of long hours in the saddle. For some people it might be getting out of their comfort zone and riding the zip lines in the jungles of Costa Rica or hiking the red rocks of Sedona to see the ancient native cave drawings. None of these would have been possible were it not for the work, the physical effort, expended to grasp the reward.

For me, it's been learning to climb cliffs and rocks, despite my arthritis. I even climbed a waterfall in Australia—well, not the waterfall itself but the rocks all around it. Some of my friends think I'm too much of a physical risk-taker. They'll say, "Patch, you've got arthritis and you're going heli-skiing?" And I say, "Sure, why not?"

I know that most of the time I talk about moderation in physical activity and that's certainly the crux of my message. You have to be very real about physical activity and that means doing what works for *you* and not stressing yourself out over it.

But sometimes there's the special physical activity, the one that pushes you just a little further. You get through it and you think, "Hey, I really did that!" One of my staff members, Rod, has fought to keep his weight down and is now in very good shape. To help others and encourage himself, he pushed himself to do an incredible bike trek across Canada in support of cancer research for children. The neat thing about doing the physical activity that pushes you a bit is that it's immediate. You have to be so completely in the present moment. It's not like running a business, where you have meetings and constantly plan ahead. It's not like taking your favorite route downtown and knowing it off by heart. It's about being keenly in the now. In fact, that's where all exercise happens. By engaging your body, you're in the now. And when you are present and in the moment, your learning curve is dramatic.

One of the most interesting learning curves I experienced was horseback riding. Off and on through my life I'd ridden a little, Western-style, but horses for the most part were not on my radar—until my daughter Tygre wanted to learn to ride English-style at the age of six. So we took lessons that summer because I figured it would be better to do it together rather than with me just watching. We rode for three years and then I got us some inexpensive horses when she turned nine (however, nothing else about horses is inexpensive!). The great thing is, now I am able to include my other daughter Kilee, who is autistic. You gotta just laugh sometimes about the way things work out. For Kilee, it's been a very liberating experience.

So you might think to yourself, "Hey, that guy's in his fifties. Why does he need to learn to ride English?" Well, because the process of learning how to do something new, outside of your comfort zone, teaches you other things. It teaches you alertness—to notice things in the environment you haven't noticed before. You learn to grow, adapt, and, in the process, you stay young! It teaches you to breathe more deeply: it teaches your brain to lay down new pathways of skill.

That's the absolute best thing about exercise—it makes so many other things possible, things you've always wanted to do just for the heck of it. It makes your life experience richer and gives you great stories to tell.

DO THIS

After you've been physically active for a while, think about trying something that might be just a bit outside your comfort zone. It doesn't have to be dangerous. It could be learning to dance the tango or hiking all the way to the bottom of the Grand Canyon (and back up again, don't forget that!) or going sea kayaking in ocean swells, or following the walking path of the North American explorers—so many possibilities.

NOW THAT YOU'VE GOT THE BIG PICTURE, HERE'S A BIGGER ONE

When people first start an exercise regimen, they often judge themselves harshly. They focus on their short-comings or on how far they have to go, rather than congratulating themselves for showing up, seeing the great gift they have given to themselves, and acknowledging how far they have come.

I have found that exercise has not only been a source of physical joy, but it has provided me with moments of spiritual connection as well. I have frequently said that your body will thank you for exercising—you'll have more energy than you've ever had before and your body will feel fantastic. Sometimes you get an even better surprise—the gift of feeling that your mind, heart, spirit, and body are truly one.

A few years ago I went climbing by myself in Palm Springs. I had noticed some small mountains nearby.

I hadn't done any serious climbing since I got arthritis, but they didn't look that high. I left the hotel at 5:30 a.m. and began the climb. It was much steeper than I had thought, and before long I was clambering over rocks and boulders, wondering what on earth I was trying to prove—it was like being on nature's StairMaster. The sun was rising behind me when all of a sudden I saw something glinting higher up.

A coyote was looking down at me from seventy-five feet (twenty-three meters) above. The sunlight had caught the edge of its fur and made it shine golden. It was the most beautiful sight. The backdrop of the mountains, the sunrise, and this breathtaking animal so close to me made me speechless. I felt something I can only describe as awe. I was keenly aware of my breathing, my muscles, my beating heart, and the stillness of nature all around me. I would never have experienced this if I hadn't pushed myself to try that climb. On my way back down the mountain, there were two more coyotes, watching me from a safe distance.

I was back for breakfast at 9 a.m. Do you think the other hotel guests had any clue about what I had just enjoyed? Two days after I saw the coyotes, I climbed up the gondola hill in Palm Springs and did my very first overhang—scary, challenging, and rewarding. I can still remember the feeling of accomplishment and that keen, clear sense of being alive.

A lot of self-help methods are based on mental discipline or on working through emotional issues. What these approaches lack is an awareness of how the body is an integral part of the equation. The health of your body influences what you experience in your mind. There is no split. If you can engage your whole spirit in the pursuit of fitness—not just your intellect, not just your emotions—but instead everything inside you that is truly *you*, you'll discover what it is to be a whole person.

Your body needs and wants exercise. Your mind needs exercise. Your heart (the loving part of you) needs exercise. Your spirit needs exercise. All aspects of you live within your body. All these parts of you allow your soul to be free because when your body, mind, heart, and spirit are in sync, you resonate with life itself. You really can experience fitness for the soul.

PRESENT PERFECT

There is only one point of perfection that's always there for us—the present moment. All the energy you will ever need is right here in the present. It's not in the past or the future. Right here and now there is a really big present waiting for you. This present will help you be incredibly successful. This present will make your day more fun. This present will make your whole life better!

How do we get the present? How do we improve the look, feel, taste, smell, and experience of our life? We are going to live and breathe happiness. I believe true happiness comes from living in the present. My grandmother used to say, "Don't replay all the day's trivialities and irritations in your mind before bed." I say, "Don't watch the late-night news! Instead, feel gratitude for today's happy moments."

Spiritual teachers say that "being in the now" is the path to enlightenment. I think that's true. On a lighter note, it's also sexy! If you're a person whose entire energy is concentrated in the present moment, if you're a person who is really *right there* and not off somewhere else in your mind, you'll attract so many great things in your life. That's smart! Exercise can help you experience that state. Give your body what it needs and it will give back to you. That's strong!

Say *yes* to the healthy you! To the sexy you! To the smart you! To the strong you! Say *yes* to your life!

ACKNOWLEDGMENTS

First of all, I would like to acknowledge all the wonderful members of my GoodLife Clubs who have made physical activity a regular part of their lives. Daily they experience the energy boost, productivity, positive attitude, and vitality that only exercise can provide. I am grateful also to the GoodLife staff in all 200 clubs (opened, in-the-works, or planned), whose hard work and dedication make it possible for members to feel the joy of exercise.

I would like to recognize Jane Riddell, my second-in-command at GoodLife since it started thirty years ago, and every fabulous member of the executive team at GoodLife. Jane's intelligence, loyalty, and the love of fitness which she exemplifies in her own life, have always been an inspiration to me.

To Dorothy, my almost 90-year-old mom, who still works daily with the company. She is her own very "real" sexy, smart, and strong.

To Megan Cameron, GoodLife's Director of Public Relations, my deepest gratitude and appreciation for all the wonderful things you do to assist me in communicating with the public. Your commitment to this book has played a huge role in helping it reach many thousands of readers.

To Sharon Lindenburger, my "scribe," who as a skilled journalist and writer so deftly rendered my words and thoughts onto the printed page.

To my agent, Cathy Hemming, who so strongly believed in this project and brought me to an excellent publisher.

To my publisher, John Wiley and Sons: it has been a tremendous experience working with you. Leah Fairbank is a wonderfully sensitive and affirming editor who made it easy to create a book I am proud of. Thanks also to editor Abigail Rasminsky for asking us some hard questions and requesting clarifications that resulted in us honing the focus of the book to directly speak to where readers are at.

Finally, I wish to acknowledge you, the reader. It gives me great pleasure that you have picked up this book. No matter where you are in your life right now, it is my hope that the suggestions and encouragement you find here will inspire you to know that you can be sexy, smart, and strong, whether you're 18 or 80!

David Patchell-Evans ("Patch")